~DietMinder~

Personal
Food & Fitness Journal

by MemoryMinder Journals, Inc.

"Your Key to Success!"

This journal belongs to

_____

_____

MemoryMinder Journals, Inc. makes no claims whatsoever regarding the interpretation or utilization of any information contained herein and/or recorded by the user of this journal.

DietMinder *Personal Food & Fitness Journal*
MemoryMinder Journals, Inc.
by F. and D. Wilkins
Original Copyrights ©1997, ©2000
2012-2013 Edition

ISBN# 978-0-9637968-3-7
UPC 7-00703-81836-9

For information regarding this publication contact:
MemoryMinder Journals, Inc.
P.O. Box 23108
Eugene, OR 97402-0425
(541)342-2300

Printed and assembled in the USA

*It's been proven time and again...
people who write down what they
eat and drink have greater success
losing weight than those who don't.*

~Contents~

~*Introduction*~

Here's a food and fitness diary that works with virtually *any* plan! Whatever your goal, whatever your program, this is the book for you. The **DietMinder** *Personal Food & Fitness Journal* was designed to help you succeed by focusing on your goals and keeping track of your efforts. It's that simple.

You'll be amazed to find how writing in your **DietMinder** will help. After recording the details of just one day, you'll suddenly become more committed to your objectives and develop a new level of awareness. As the days go by, seeing your hard work and accomplishments in black and white will give you the motivation you need to carry on. (Don't worry if you falter now and then, just be sure to write it down. A little bit of healthy guilt can work wonders!)

As you write in your **DietMinder** you'll create a record of what works best for you. If your first program does not prove satisfactory, you'll have your own record to challenge or improve upon the next time. (Over ninety daily two-page sets are provided for three months of steady dieting or for several shorter sessions.)

It is our hope that you'll enjoy using your **DietMinder** and that it will lead you on the road to a lasting lifestyle of healthy eating and regular exercise. Some of the changes in this edition are the result of comments from professional fitness experts as well as from people who have used previous versions. We sincerely appreciate those kind suggestions and, as before, welcome any new comments you may have.

~Tips for Using Your~
DietMinder

The **DietMinder** *Personal Food & Fitness Journal* is so easy to use it hardly needs instructions. But, if you take just a few moments to review the following tips, it will help you get the maximum benefit.*

You'll need a handbook of food counts for recording foods that don't have labels and foods not already listed in the back of the **DietMinder**. The internet can provide this information as well.

The **DietMinder** consists of three sections. The cream-colored pages make it easy to differentiate between these sections which are listed accordingly in the Table of Contents. The following paragraphs explain each page in detail.

1 *Personal Goals...* Define your goals and how you plan to attain them. This is an important first step. (Three of these two-page sets are provided in case you use your journal for more than one diet.)

2 *Daily Targets...* Fill in the boxes with your food and activity goals. It's not necessary to fill in every box...just those that pertain to your own plan. The "Daily Food Targets" boxes relate directly to the "Grand Totals" boxes on the daily pages.

3 *Statistics...* List your measurements and readings before you begin so you can measure and compare results as you progress. Again, just fill in the blanks which pertain to your own plan and goals.

4 *Photo Page...* Paste your picture(s) here for added motivation. If you prefer, this space can be used for diet instructions, workout schedules, or whatever reference you might find useful.

Be sure to consult your physician before making any significant changes in diet or exercise.

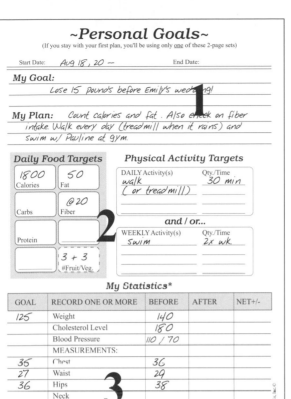

~Personal Goals~
(If you stay with your first plan, you'll be using only <u>one</u> of these 2-page sets)

Start Date: _Aug 18, 20 —_   End Date: _____

My Goal:
Lose 15 pounds before Emily's wedding!

My Plan:
Count calories and fat. Also check on fiber intake. Walk every day (treadmill when it rains) and swim w/ Pauline at gym.

Daily Food Targets

1800 Calories	**50** Fat
Carbs	**@ 20** Fiber
Protein	
	3 + 3 #Fruit/Veg.

Physical Activity Targets

DAILY Activity(s) — Qty./Time
walk — _30 min_
(or treadmill)

and / or...

WEEKLY Activity(s) — Qty./Time
swim — _2x wk_

My Statistics*

GOAL	RECORD ONE OR MORE	BEFORE	AFTER	NET+/-
_125_	Weight	_140_		
	Cholesterol Level	_180_		
	Blood Pressure	_110 / 70_		
	MEASUREMENTS:			
_35_	Chest	_36_		
_27_	Waist	_29_		
_36_	Hips	_38_		
	Neck			
	Upper Arms			
_22_	Thighs	_23_		
	Calves			

*See back of book for related "Weekly Progress" chart

MemoryMinder Journals, Inc.©

Goals & Statistics

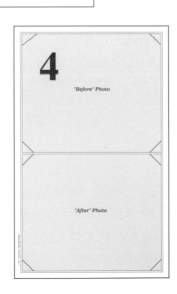

"Before" Photo

"After" Photo

Photos or ???

Food or Beverage (left daily page)... Start each day by posting the date and day number. On the days you step on the scale (morning weigh-ins are best), write your weight in the box provided. Throughout the day, list everything you eat or drink and the serving size, no matter how small the portion. Make note of the time meals are eaten. Try to write down your foods within fifteen minutes of eating so you won't forget.

Food Counts & more (l. & r. pages)... Seven columns are provided (five pre-labeled, two for any other count of your choice). Each meal's title bar can be used to note details such as where you ate, sugar reading, etc. Water can be monitored in the check-off boxes. *It's not necessary to fill in all the columns and spaces; use only those which pertain to your own plan.*

Day # 3	Wednesday August 19, 20— Day of the Week & Date			Weight: 138	Time 7AM

FOOD OR BEVERAGE — 5 — Calories / Fat grams / Carbs/gms / Fiber/gms / Protein/gms

BREAKFAST	Amount	Calories	Fat grams	Carbs/gms	Fiber/gms	Protein/gms
Oatmeal	1 c	150	3		4	
1% milk	1 c	110	2.5		0	
Or Juice	6 oz	90	0		0	
Coffee	2 c	10	0		0	
Time: 7:30 Breakfast Totals >		360	5.5		4	

SNACK	Amount					
Muffin	1	70	1		1.4	
Jelly	1 Tb	60	0		0	
Time: 9:30 Snack Totals >		130	1		1.4	

LUNCH	Amount	(Lunch w/ Joni & Mary)				
Salad	1 c	25	0		1	
Apple	1	81	0		3.7	
Ranch dres.	1 Tb	70	7		0	
Ham sand.	1/2	210	10		1	
Iced tea	12 oz	2	0		0	
Time: 12:30 Lunch Totals >		388	17		5.7	

SNACK	Amount					
Almonds	14	85	8		1.5	
Grapes	10	36	.3		3	
Diet soda	1	0	0		0	
Time: 4:00 Snack Totals >		121	8.3		1.8	
PAGE SUBTOTALS:		999	31.8		12.9	

Memory-Minder Journals, Inc ©

Food & Beverages (left page)

Daily Grand Totals (right daily page)... After your last meal or snack of the day, use the area provided to "do the math" and enter the grand totals in the appropriate boxes. For added good health, use the dotted-line box to record your number of servings of fruits and vegetables.

8 *Vitamins, Supplements, Meds...* List any vitamins, herbs, other diet supplements, and medications you took today. You can also note the time of day you took them. This information may be useful for future reference.

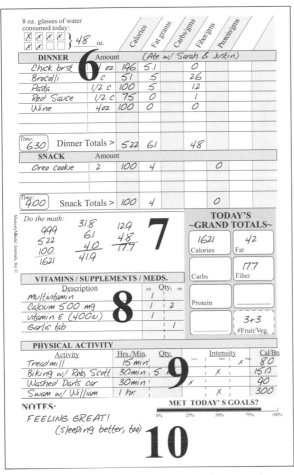

Totals, exercise, etc. (right page)

9 *Physical Activity* ... List your activities for the day and the amount of time you spent doing them. In addition to hours and minutes, your activities can be measured by the "quantity" of units completed such as laps, miles, etc. Intensity level may also be noted as well as the approximate calories burned (Cal/Bn).

10 *Notes area...* Use the bar graph to record how well you did at reaching today's goals, then briefly summarize your day. Are you feeling good? Depressed? Energetic? Are you making progress? What was your high or low point today? (Keep other statistics of your progress in the back of your **DietMinder**. See Tips 12 and 13.)

Facts... (See alphabetically tabbed pages in the back of the book.) Use this section to create your own handy reference guide for the foods you eat most often. Over one hundred common foods are already listed. If you calculate the counts for your favorite food combinations (such as casseroles, sandwiches, etc.) and post them here, you'll be able to save time when filling out the Daily Pages.

Favorite Foods Facts
continued

~FOOD OR BEVERAGE~	AMT.	Calories	Fat grams	Carbs/gms	Fiber/gms	Protein/gms
M						
Mac.& Cheese, *Kraft*	1 c.	410	18.5	48.0	1.0	11.0
Maple syrup	1T.	50	0	13.0	0	0
Margarine	1T.	100	11.0	0	0	0
Mayonnaise, *Best F*	1	100	11.00	0	0	0
Milk, whole	1	150	8.2	11.4	0	8.0
Milk, non-fat	1	90	0	13.0	0	9.0
Muffin, English	1	132	1.0	28.7	2.6	4.6
Mushroom, raw	1/2 c.	9	.2	1.6	.4	.7
Mustard	1T.	11	1.0	1.0	0	1.0
meatloaf	4 oz.	300	21	0	0	28
muffin, Bluberry	1	130	5	18	1	2
michelle's quiche	1 sl.	320	10	3	1	10
N-O	AMT.					
Nectarine, medium	1	67	.6	16.0	2.2	1.3
Noodles, egg, cooked	1 c.	212	2.4	39.7	1.8	7.6
Oatmeal, dry	1/2 c.	150	3.0	27.0	4.0	5.0
Olive oil	1Tb.	120	14.0	0	0	0
Onion, raw, chopped	1/2 c.	30	.1	6.9	1.4	.9
Orange, navel	1	65	.1	16.3	3.4	1.4
Orange juice	6 oz.	80	0	20.0	.1	0
Oysters, raw	6	57	21	33	0	59

Favorite Foods Facts

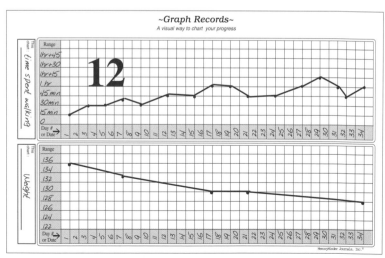

Graph Records (see next page)

12 *Graph Records...* Plotting your achievements on a graph is one way to chart your progress. Sometimes a picture is worth a thousand words! Following the "Favorite Foods Facts" are four graphs. These can be used to chart progress and/or compare activities with results. (For our example, we compared walking time with weight loss.) This is an option, of course.

13 *Weekly Progress...* Following the Graph Records is a chart that relates directly to the statistics list in the Goals Section. This can be updated weekly or whenever you desire by simply entering the date and the measurements or readings of your choice.

~Weekly Progress~					
DATES:	Aug 18	Aug 25			
Weight	140	136			
Cholesterol Level	180	-			
Blood Pressure	110/70	110/65			
MEASUREMENTS:					
Chest	36	36			
Waist	29	28			
Hips	38	37.5			
Neck					
Upper Arms					
Thighs	23	23			
Calves					
DATES:					
Weight					
Cholesterol Level					
Blood Pressure					
MEASUREMENTS:					
Chest					
Waist					
Hips					
Neck					
Upper Arms					
Thighs					
Calves					
DATES:					
Weight					
Cholesterol Level					
Blood Pressure					
MEASUREMENTS:					
Chest					
Waist					
Hips					
Neck					
Upper Arms					
Thighs					
Calves					

Weekly Progress

The **DietMinder** also includes a reference calendar, a re-order form, and a handy vinyl utility pocket which can be used to hold recipes, diet instructions, health club cards, workout schedules, etc.

Another option... If you wish, the daily pages of your Journal can be used as a meal planner. Simply pencil in your planned food and beverages with their corresponding counts. After meals, highlight or place a check mark by the foods you actually ate and calculate only those figures.

Remember, the **DietMinder** is designed to work with virtually *any* food and fitness plan. Take it with you wherever you go... it's conveniently sized for home, work or travel. If you use your Journal faithfully, your commitment will be strong and your goals will soon be reached!

~Information on the Web~

The internet sites listed here can provide a wealth of information regarding food, health, diets, and more. However, information found on any website should never be a substitute for professional medical advice or treatment.

These sites are listed solely for your convenience and only to heighten your awareness of health and fitness, not to suggest or recommend any given treatment, product, or action.

Always consult your doctor before making any significant change in your diet, exercise, or other health practices.

www.Nutrition.gov
This huge site contains national resource information
from the federal government.

www.Prevention.com
The *Prevention* magazines are popular sources
for health and fitness news.

www.RealAge.com
Online home of the YOU Docs. This site features the
popular RealAge Test, the Docs Daily Blog and much more!

www.CalorieLab.com
This site includes a free search feature for finding
the calorie content in thousands of foods.

www.KidsHealth.org
Devoted to improving the health of children, this is
three sites in one for Parents, Kids, and Teens

www.EveryDiet.org
This site contains a compilation of information
on a multitude of diet plans

Realize.com
When looking for information pertaining to
bariatric surgery options & procedures, this site may be helpful.

www.ConsumerReports.org
Click on the "health" tab for impartial reviews on diets, nutrition,
exercise equipment, home medical supplies, safety, and more.

www.MemoryMinder.com
View our journal pages, read reviews, link to online bookstores
or use the "direct from publisher" order form.

Two Ways to Measure Weight

1. BMI (Body Mass Index)

In this method your BMI number is calculated in a formula which then relates to a standard BMI Chart. The formula is:

Weight (lb) ÷ [Height (inches)]^2 x 703 = BMI number
Example: Weight = 150 lbs, height = 5'5" (65")
Calculation: [150 ÷ (65)^2] x 703 = 24.96
(The metric formula is weight (kg) ÷ [height (m)]^2)

BMI	Weight Status
Below 18.5	Underweight
18.5 - 24.9	Normal
25.0 - 29.9	Overweight
30.0 & over	Obese

2. Standard Adult Height/Weight Tables

In this method healthy weight has been determined using statistics from insurance industry mortality tables. (Based on body frame size.)

	WOMEN				MEN		
Height	Small	Med.	Large	Height	Small	Med.	Large
4'10"	102-111	109-121	118-131	5'2"	128-134	131-141	138-150
4'11"	103-113	111-123	120-134	5'3"	130-136	133-143	140-153
5'0"	104-115	113-126	122-137	5'4"	132-138	135-145	142-156
5'1"	106-118	115-129	125-140	5'5"	134-140	137-148	144-160
5'2"	108-121	118-132	128-143	5'6"	136-142	139-151	146-164
5'3"	111-124	121-135	131-147	5'7"	138-145	142-154	149-168
5'4"	114-127	124-138	134-151	5'8"	140-148	145-157	152-172
5'5"	117-130	127-141	137-155	5'9"	142-151	148-160	155-176
5'6"	120-133	130-144	140-159	5'10"	144-154	151-163	158-180
5'7"	123-136	133-147	143-163	5'11"	146-157	154-166	161-184
5'8"	126-139	136-150	146-167	6'0"	149-160	157-170	164-188
5'9"	129-142	139-153	149-170	6'1"	152-164	160-174	168-192
5'10"	132-145	142-156	152-173	6'2"	155-168	164-178	172-197
5'11"	135-148	145-159	155-176	6'3"	158-172	167-182	176-202
6'0"	138-151	148-162	158-179	6'4"	162-176	171-187	181-207

~Useful Tidbits~

Serving Sizes

What counts as an "average serving"?

Grains: 1 slice bread, 1 oz. ready-to-eat cereal, ½ cup cooked cereal, rice or pasta

Vegetables: 1 cup raw leafy veg., ½ cup other veg. cooked or raw, ¾ cup veg. juice

Fruits: 1 med. apple, banana or orange, ½ cup chopped, cooked or canned fruit, ¾ cup fruit juice

Milk Group: 1 cup milk or yogurt, 1½ oz. natural cheese, 2 oz. processed cheese

Meat & Beans, etc.: 2-3 oz. cooked lean meat, poultry or fish, 1/3 cup nuts, 1/2 cup dried beans

Heart Rates

Ideal heart rate during aerobic exercise

(bpm = beats per minute)

AGE	Ideal rate
20	100-170 bpm
25	98-166 bpm
30	95-162 bpm
35	93-157 bpm
40	90-153 bpm
45	88-149 bpm
50	85-145 bpm
55	83-140 bpm
60	80-136 bpm
65	78-132 bpm
70	75-128 bpm

Calorie Expenditure Guide

The rate at which your body burns calories is determined by your weight and by the intensity of your physical activity. The more you weigh and/or the harder you work, the more calories you will burn per hour. So true caloric expenditure can vary significantly from person to person.

These activities burn roughly 150 calories:*

- Walking 2 miles in **30** minutes
- Gardening for **30-45** minutes
- Raking leaves for **30** minutes
- Pushing a stroller 1.5 miles in **30** minutes
- Dancing fast for **30** minutes
- Bicycling 5 miles in **30** minutes
- Running 1.5 miles in **15** minutes
- Stairwalking for **15** minutes
- Playing basketball for **15-20** minutes
- Swimming laps for **20** minutes
- Jumping rope for **15** minutes
- Shoveling snow for **15** minutes

*Burning approximately 150 calories per day engaged in physical activity is considered "moderate activity."

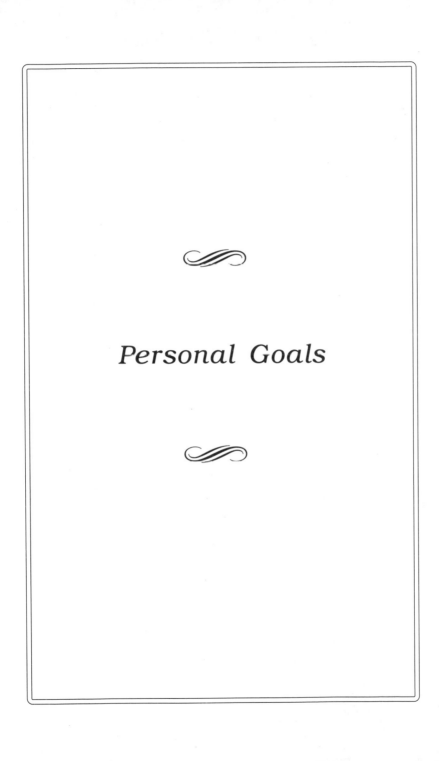

Personal Goals

~Personal Goals~

(If you stay with your first plan, you'll be using only <u>one</u> of these 2-page sets)

Start Date: _____   End Date: _____

My Goal:

_____

_____

My Plan:

_____

_____

Daily Food Targets

Calories	Fat
Carbs	Fiber
Protein	_____
_____	#Fruit/Veg.

Physical Activity Targets

DAILY Activity(s)	Qty./Time
_____	_____
_____	_____
_____	_____

and / or...

WEEKLY Activity(s)	Qty./Time
_____	_____
_____	_____
_____	_____

My Statistics*

GOAL	RECORD ONE OR MORE	BEFORE	AFTER	NET+/-
	Weight			
	Cholesterol Level			
	Blood Pressure			
	MEASUREMENTS:			
	Chest			
	Waist			
	Hips			
	Neck			
	Upper Arms			
	Thighs			
	Calves			

*See back of book for related "Weekly Progress" chart

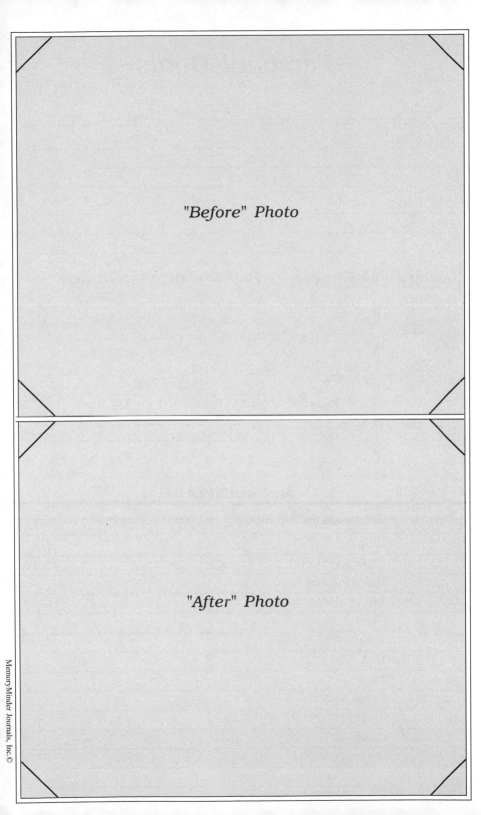

"*Before*" Photo

"*After*" Photo

~Personal Goals~

(If you stay with your first plan, you'll be using only <u>one</u> of these 2-page sets)

Start Date: _____   End Date: _____

My Goal: _____
_____
_____

My Plan: _____
_____
_____

Daily Food Targets

Calories	Fat
Carbs	Fiber
Protein	_____
_____	#Fruit/Veg.

Physical Activity Targets

DAILY Activity(s)	Qty./Time
_____	_____
_____	_____
_____	_____

and / or...

WEEKLY Activity(s)	Qty./Time
_____	_____
_____	_____
_____	_____

My Statistics*

GOAL	RECORD ONE OR MORE	BEFORE	AFTER	NET+/-
	Weight			
	Cholesterol Level			
	Blood Pressure			
	MEASUREMENTS:			
	Chest			
	Waist			
	Hips			
	Neck			
	Upper Arms			
	Thighs			
	Calves			

*See back of book for related "Weekly Progress" chart

MemoryMinder Journals, Inc.©

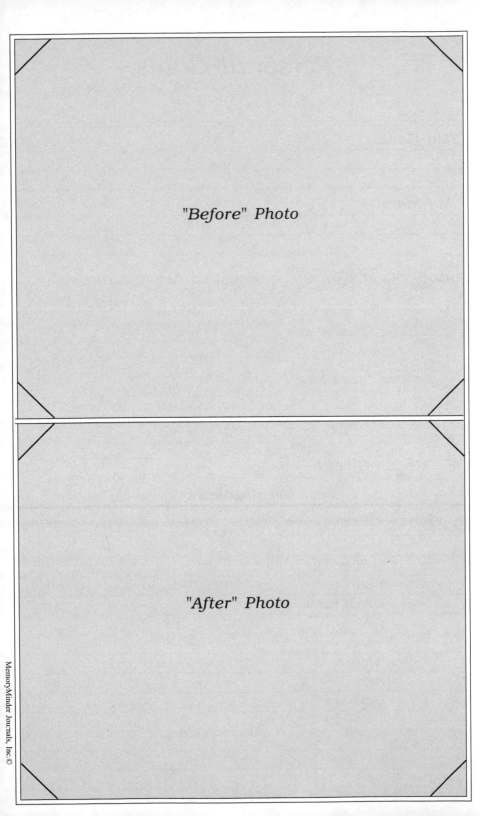

"Before" Photo

"After" Photo

~Personal Goals~

(If you stay with your first plan, you'll be using only <u>one</u> of these 2-page sets)

Start Date: _____   End Date: _____

My Goal: _____

_____

My Plan: _____

_____

Daily Food Targets

Calories	Fat
Carbs	Fiber
Protein	
	#Fruit/Veg.

Physical Activity Targets

DAILY Activity(s)	Qty./Time
_____	_____
_____	_____
_____	_____

and / or...

WEEKLY Activity(s)	Qty./Time
_____	_____
_____	_____
_____	_____

My Statistics*

GOAL	RECORD ONE OR MORE	BEFORE	AFTER	NET+/-
	Weight			
	Cholesterol Level			
	Blood Pressure			
	MEASUREMENTS:			
	Chest			
	Waist			
	Hips			
	Neck			
	Upper Arms			
	Thighs			
	Calves			

*See back of book for related "Weekly Progress" chart

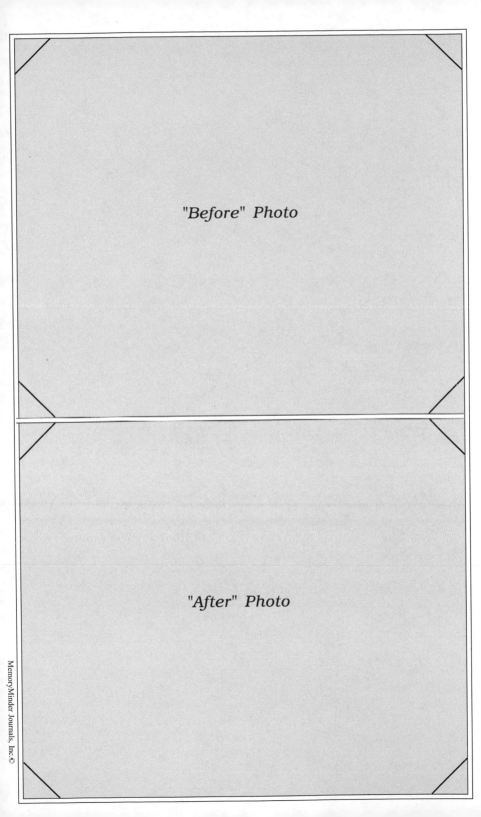

"Before" Photo

"After" Photo

Daily Food
&
Fitness Records

Day #		Weight:	
			Time

Day of the Week & Date

FOOD OR BEVERAGE		Calories	Fat grams	Carbs/gms	Fiber/gms	Protein/gms		
BREAKFAST	Amount							
Time: Breakfast Totals >								
SNACK	Amount							
Time: Snack Totals >								
LUNCH	Amount							
Time: Lunch Totals >								
SNACK	Amount							
Time: Snack Totals >								
PAGE SUBTOTALS:								

8 oz. glasses of water
consumed today:

} _____ oz.

	Calories	Fat grams	Carbs/gms	Fiber/gms	Protein/gms	
DINNER Amount						
Time: Dinner Totals >						
SNACK Amount						
Time: Snack Totals >						

Do the math:

TODAY'S ~GRAND TOTALS~

Calories	Fat
Carbs	Fiber
Protein	
	#Fruit/Veg.

VITAMINS / SUPPLEMENTS / MEDS.

Description	AM Qty. PM

PHYSICAL ACTIVITY

Activity	Hrs./Min.	Qty.	Intensity			Cal/Bn
			Low	Med.	High	

NOTES:

MET TODAY'S GOALS?

0%　　25%　　50%　　75%　　100%

Day #							Weight:		Time

Day of the Week & Date

FOOD OR BEVERAGE		Calories	Fat grams	Carbs/gms	Fiber/gms	Protein/gms	
BREAKFAST	Amount						
Time: Breakfast Totals >							
SNACK	Amount						
Time: Snack Totals >							
LUNCH	Amount						
Time: Lunch Totals >							
SNACK	Amount						
Time: Snack Totals >							
PAGE SUBTOTALS:							

8 oz. glasses of water
consumed today:

☐ ☐ ☐
☐ ☐ ☐ } _____ oz.

		Calories	Fat grams	Carbs/gms	Fiber/gms	Protein/gms	
DINNER	Amount						
Time:	Dinner Totals >						
SNACK	Amount						
Time:	Snack Totals >						

Do the math:

TODAY'S ~GRAND TOTALS~

Calories	Fat
Carbs	Fiber
Protein	_____
_____	#Fruit/Veg.

VITAMINS / SUPPLEMENTS / MEDS.

Description	AM Qty. PM

PHYSICAL ACTIVITY

Activity	Hrs./Min.	Qty.	Intensity (Low / Med. / High)	Cal/Bn

NOTES:

MET TODAY'S GOALS?

| 0% | 25% | 50% | 75% | 100% |

Day #							Weight:	Time

Day of the Week & Date

FOOD OR BEVERAGE	Calories	Fat grams	Carbs/gms	Fiber/gms	Protein/gms	
BREAKFAST Amount						
Time: Breakfast Totals >						
SNACK Amount						
Time: Snack Totals >						
LUNCH Amount						
Time: Lunch Totals >						
SNACK Amount						
Time: Snack Totals >						
PAGE SUBTOTALS:						

8 oz. glasses of water consumed today:

☐ ☐ ☐ ☐
☐ ☐ ☐ ☐ } _____ oz.

		Calories	Fat grams	Carbs/gms	Fiber/gms	Protein/gms	
DINNER	Amount						
Time:	Dinner Totals >						
SNACK	Amount						
Time:	Snack Totals >						

Do the math:

TODAY'S ~GRAND TOTALS~

Calories	Fat
Carbs	Fiber
Protein	
	#Fruit/Veg.

VITAMINS / SUPPLEMENTS / MEDS.

Description	AM	Qty.	PM

PHYSICAL ACTIVITY

Activity	Hrs./Min.	Qty.	Intensity Low / Med. / High	Cal/Bn

NOTES:

MET TODAY'S GOALS?

0%	25%	50%	75%	100%

Day #			Weight:	
	Day of the Week & Date			*Time*

FOOD OR BEVERAGE		Calories	Fat grams	Carbs/gms	Fiber/gms	Protein/gms		
BREAKFAST	Amount							
Time: Breakfast Totals >								
SNACK	Amount							
Time: Snack Totals >								
LUNCH	Amount							
Time: Lunch Totals >								
SNACK	Amount							
Time: Snack Totals >								
PAGE SUBTOTALS:								

8 oz. glasses of water
consumed today:
☐ ☐ ☐ ☐
☐ ☐ ☐ ☐ } _____ oz.

		Calories	Fat grams	Carbs/gms	Fiber/gms	Protein/gms	
DINNER	Amount						
Time: Dinner Totals >							
SNACK	Amount						
Time: Snack Totals >							

Do the math:

TODAY'S ~GRAND TOTALS~

Calories Fat

Carbs Fiber

Protein _____

_____ #Fruit/Veg.

VITAMINS / SUPPLEMENTS / MEDS.

Description	AM Qty. PM

PHYSICAL ACTIVITY

Activity	Hrs./Min.	Qty.	Intensity (Low / Med. / High)	Cal/Bn

NOTES:

MET TODAY'S GOALS?

0%   25%   50%   75%   100%

Day #							Weight:	
								Time

Day of the Week & Date

FOOD OR BEVERAGE		*Calories*	*Fat grams*	*Carbs/gms*	*Fiber/gms*	*Protein/gms*		
BREAKFAST	Amount							
Time: Breakfast Totals >								
SNACK	Amount							
Time: Snack Totals >								
LUNCH	Amount							
Time: Lunch Totals >								
SNACK	Amount							
Time: Snack Totals >								
PAGE SUBTOTALS:								

8 oz. glasses of water consumed today:

☐☐☐☐
☐☐☐☐ } _____ oz.

		Calories	Fat grams	Carbs/gms	Fiber/gms	Protein/gms	
DINNER	Amount						
Time: [ ] Dinner Totals >							
SNACK	Amount						
Time: [ ] Snack Totals >							

Do the math:

TODAY'S ~GRAND TOTALS~

Calories	Fat
Carbs	Fiber
Protein	_____
_____	#Fruit/Veg.

VITAMINS/SUPPLEMENTS/MEDS.

Description	AM Qty. PM

PHYSICAL ACTIVITY

Activity	Hrs./Min.	Qty.	Intensity (Low / Med. / High)	Cal/Bn

NOTES:

MET TODAY'S GOALS?

0%   25%   50%   75%   100%

MemoryMinder Journals, Inc. ©

Weight:

Time

Day of the Week & Date

FOOD OR BEVERAGE		Calories	Fat grams	Carbs/gms	Fiber/gms	Protein/gms	
BREAKFAST	Amount						
Time: Breakfast Totals >							
SNACK	Amount						
Time: Snack Totals >							
LUNCH	Amount						
Time: Lunch Totals >							
SNACK	Amount						
Time: Snack Totals >							
PAGE SUBTOTALS:							

8 oz. glasses of water
consumed today:

☐ ☐ ☐ ☐
☐ ☐ ☐ ☐ } _____ oz.

	Calories	Fat grams	Carbs/gms	Fiber/gms	Protein/gms	
DINNER Amount						
Time:						
Dinner Totals >						
SNACK Amount						
Time:						
Snack Totals >						

Do the math:

TODAY'S ~GRAND TOTALS~

Calories	Fat
Carbs	Fiber
Protein	
	#Fruit/Veg.

VITAMINS / SUPPLEMENTS / MEDS.

Description	AM	Qty.	PM

PHYSICAL ACTIVITY

Activity	Hrs./Min.	Qty.	Intensity			Cal/Bn
			Low	Med.	High	

NOTES:

MET TODAY'S GOALS?

| 0% | 25% | 50% | 75% | 100% |

| Day # | | | | | | | Weight: | | Time | |

Day of the Week & Date

FOOD OR BEVERAGE	Amount	Calories	Fat grams	Carbs/gms	Fiber/gms	Protein/gms		
BREAKFAST	Amount							
Time: Breakfast Totals >								
SNACK	Amount							
Time: Snack Totals >								
LUNCH	Amount							
Time: Lunch Totals >								
SNACK	Amount							
Time: Snack Totals >								
PAGE SUBTOTALS:								

8 oz. glasses of water consumed today:

☐☐☐☐
☐☐☐☐ } _____ oz.

	Amount	Calories	Fat grams	Carbs/gms	Fiber/gms	Protein/gms	
DINNER							
Time: Dinner Totals >							
SNACK	Amount						
Time: Snack Totals >							

Do the math:

TODAY'S ~GRAND TOTALS~

Calories	Fat
Carbs	Fiber
Protein	
	#Fruit/Veg.

VITAMINS / SUPPLEMENTS / MEDS.

Description	AM Qty. PM

PHYSICAL ACTIVITY

Activity	Hrs./Min.	Qty.	Intensity Low / Med. / High	Cal/Bn

NOTES:

MET TODAY'S GOALS?

0%   25%   50%   75%   100%

Day #							Weight:	

Day of the Week & Date

Time

FOOD OR BEVERAGE		Calories	Fat grams	Carbs/gms	Fiber/gms	Protein/gms	
BREAKFAST	Amount						
Time: Breakfast Totals >							
SNACK	Amount						
Time: Snack Totals >							
LUNCH	Amount						
Time: Lunch Totals >							
SNACK	Amount						
Time: Snack Totals >							
PAGE SUBTOTALS:							

8 oz. glasses of water
consumed today:

☐ ☐ ☐
☐ ☐ ☐ } _____ oz.

	Calories	Fat grams	Carbs/gms	Fiber/gms	Protein/gms	
DINNER Amount						
Time: Dinner Totals >						
SNACK Amount						
Time: Snack Totals >						

Do the math:

TODAY'S ~GRAND TOTALS~

Calories

Fat

Carbs

Fiber

Protein

_____

_____   #Fruit/Veg.

VITAMINS / SUPPLEMENTS / MEDS.

Description	AM Qty. PM

PHYSICAL ACTIVITY

Activity	Hrs./Min.	Qty.	Intensity Low / Med. / High	Cal/Bn

NOTES:

MET TODAY'S GOALS?

0%   25%   50%   75%   100%

Day #						Weight:	Time

Day of the Week & Date

FOOD OR BEVERAGE		Calories	Fat grams	Carbs/gms	Fiber/gms	Protein/gms	
BREAKFAST	Amount						
Time: Breakfast Totals >							
SNACK	Amount						
Time: Snack Totals >							
LUNCH	Amount						
Time: Lunch Totals >							
SNACK	Amount						
Time: Snack Totals >							
PAGE SUBTOTALS:							

MemoryMinder Journals, Inc.©

8 oz. glasses of water
consumed today:

☐ ☐ ☐
☐ ☐ ☐ } _____ oz.

	Amount	Calories	Fat grams	Carbs/gms	Fiber/gms	Protein/gms	
DINNER							
Time:	Dinner Totals >						
SNACK	Amount						
Time:	Snack Totals >						

Do the math:

TODAY'S ~GRAND TOTALS~

Calories	Fat
Carbs	Fiber
Protein	
	#Fruit/Veg.

VITAMINS / SUPPLEMENTS / MEDS.

Description	AM Qty. PM

PHYSICAL ACTIVITY

Activity	Hrs./Min.	Qty.	Intensity Low Med. High	Cal/Bn

NOTES:

MET TODAY'S GOALS?

0%   25%   50%   75%   100%

Day #				Weight:		Time

Day of the Week & Date

FOOD OR BEVERAGE		Calories	Fat grams	Carbs/gms	Fiber/gms	Protein/gms	
BREAKFAST	Amount						
Time: Breakfast Totals >							
SNACK	Amount						
Time: Snack Totals >							
LUNCH	Amount						
Time: Lunch Totals >							
SNACK	Amount						
Time: Snack Totals >							
PAGE SUBTOTALS:							

8 oz. glasses of water
consumed today:

☐ ☐ ☐ ☐
☐ ☐ ☐ } _____ oz.

		Calories	Fat grams	Carbs/gms	Fiber/gms	Protein/gms	
DINNER	Amount						
Time:	Dinner Totals >						
SNACK	Amount						
Time:	Snack Totals >						

Do the math:

TODAY'S ~GRAND TOTALS~

Calories	Fat
Carbs	Fiber
Protein	
	#Fruit/Veg.

VITAMINS / SUPPLEMENTS / MEDS.

Description	AM Qty. PM

PHYSICAL ACTIVITY

Activity	Hrs./Min.	Qty.	Intensity (Low / Med. / High)	Cal/Bn

NOTES:

MET TODAY'S GOALS?

0%   25%   50%   75%   100%

Day #			Weight:	
				Time

Day of the Week & Date

FOOD OR BEVERAGE		Calories	Fat grams	Carbs/gms	Fiber/gms	Protein/gms		
BREAKFAST	Amount							
Time: Breakfast Totals >								
SNACK	Amount							
Time: Snack Totals >								
LUNCH	Amount							
Time: Lunch Totals >								
SNACK	Amount							
Time: Snack Totals >								
PAGE SUBTOTALS:								

8 oz. glasses of water consumed today:

☐☐☐☐ } _____ oz.
☐☐☐☐

		Calories	Fat grams	Carbs/gms	Fiber/gms	Protein/gms	
DINNER	Amount						
Time:	Dinner Totals >						
SNACK	Amount						
Time:	Snack Totals >						

Do the math:

TODAY'S ~GRAND TOTALS~

Calories	Fat
Carbs	Fiber
Protein	
	#Fruit/Veg.

VITAMINS/SUPPLEMENTS/MEDS.

Description		AM Qty. PM

PHYSICAL ACTIVITY

Activity	Hrs./Min.	Qty.	Intensity (Low / Med. / High)	Cal/Bn

NOTES:

MET TODAY'S GOALS?

0%　　25%　　50%　　75%　　100%

Day of the Week & Date

FOOD OR BEVERAGE

	Amount	Calories	Fat grams	Carbs/gms	Fiber/gms	Protein/gms	
BREAKFAST							
Time: Breakfast Totals >							
SNACK							
Time: Snack Totals >							
LUNCH							
Time: Lunch Totals >							
SNACK							
Time: Snack Totals >							
PAGE SUBTOTALS:							

8 oz. glasses of water
consumed today:

☐ ☐ ☐ ☐
☐ ☐ ☐ ☐ } _____ oz.

	Calories	Fat grams	Carbs/gms	Fiber/gms	Protein/gms	
DINNER Amount						
Time: Dinner Totals >						
SNACK Amount						
Time: Snack Totals >						

Do the math:

TODAY'S ~GRAND TOTALS~

Calories	Fat

Carbs	Fiber

VITAMINS / SUPPLEMENTS / MEDS.

Description	AM Qty. PM

Protein	_____

_____	#Fruit/Veg.

PHYSICAL ACTIVITY

Activity	Hrs./Min.	Qty.	Intensity			Cal/Bn
			Low	Med.	High	

NOTES:

MET TODAY'S GOALS?

0%	25%	50%	75%	100%

Day #								Weight:		

Time

Day of the Week & Date

FOOD OR BEVERAGE		Calories	Fat grams	Carbs/gms	Fiber/gms	Protein/gms		
BREAKFAST	Amount							
Time: Breakfast Totals >								
SNACK	Amount							
Time: Snack Totals >								
LUNCH	Amount							
Time: Lunch Totals >								
SNACK	Amount							
Time: Snack Totals >								
PAGE SUBTOTALS:								

8 oz. glasses of water
consumed today:

☐ ☐ ☐ ☐
☐ ☐ ☐ ☐ } _____ oz.

		Calories	Fat grams	Carbs/gms	Fiber/gms	Protein/gms	
DINNER	Amount						
Time: Dinner Totals >							
SNACK	Amount						
Time: Snack Totals >							

Do the math:

TODAY'S ~GRAND TOTALS~

Calories	Fat
Carbs	Fiber
Protein	
	#Fruit/Veg.

VITAMINS / SUPPLEMENTS / MEDS.

Description	AM Qty. PM

PHYSICAL ACTIVITY

Activity	Hrs./Min.	Qty.	Intensity			Cal/Bn
			Low	Med.	High	

NOTES:

MET TODAY'S GOALS?

0%   25%   50%   75%   100%

Day #							Weight:	
								Time

Day of the Week & Date

FOOD OR BEVERAGE	Calories	Fat grams	Carbs/gms	Fiber/gms	Protein/gms	
BREAKFAST Amount						
Time: Breakfast Totals >						
SNACK Amount						
Time: Snack Totals >						
LUNCH Amount						
Time: Lunch Totals >						
SNACK Amount						
Time: Snack Totals >						
PAGE SUBTOTALS:						

8 oz. glasses of water
consumed today:

☐ ☐ ☐ ☐ } _____ oz.
☐ ☐ ☐ ☐

	Amount	Calories	Fat grams	Carbs/gms	Fiber/gms	Protein/gms	
DINNER							
Time: Dinner Totals >							
SNACK	Amount						
Time: Snack Totals >							

Do the math:

TODAY'S ~GRAND TOTALS~

Calories	Fat
Carbs	Fiber
Protein	
	#Fruit/Veg.

VITAMINS/SUPPLEMENTS/MEDS.

Description	AM	Qty. PM

PHYSICAL ACTIVITY

Activity	Hrs./Min.	Qty.	Intensity			Cal/Bn
			Low	Med.	High	

NOTES:

MET TODAY'S GOALS?

0%　　25%　　50%　　75%　　100%

Day #								Weight:	Time

Day of the Week & Date

FOOD OR BEVERAGE	Amount	Calories	Fat grams	Carbs/gms	Fiber/gms	Protein/gms	
BREAKFAST	Amount						
Time: Breakfast Totals >							
SNACK	Amount						
Time: Snack Totals >							
LUNCH	Amount						
Time: Lunch Totals >							
SNACK	Amount						
Time: Snack Totals >							
PAGE SUBTOTALS:							

8 oz. glasses of water consumed today: ⬚⬚⬚⬚ ⬚⬚⬚⬚ } _____ oz.

DINNER	Amount	Calories	Fat grams	Carbs/gms	Fiber/gms	Protein/gms	
Time: Dinner Totals >							

SNACK	Amount						
Time: Snack Totals >							

Do the math:

VITAMINS / SUPPLEMENTS / MEDS.

Description	AM	Qty.	PM

TODAY'S ~GRAND TOTALS~

Calories	Fat
Carbs	Fiber
Protein	
	#Fruit/Veg.

PHYSICAL ACTIVITY

Activity	Hrs./Min.	Qty.	Intensity			Cal/Bn
			Low	Med.	High	

NOTES:

MET TODAY'S GOALS?

0% 25% 50% 75% 100%

Weight:

Time

Day of the Week & Date

FOOD OR BEVERAGE	Amount	Calories	Fat grams	Carbs/gms	Fiber/gms	Protein/gms	
BREAKFAST	Amount						
Time: Breakfast Totals >							
SNACK	Amount						
Time: Snack Totals >							
LUNCH	Amount						
Time: Lunch Totals >							
SNACK	Amount						
Time: Snack Totals >							
PAGE SUBTOTALS:							

8 oz. glasses of water consumed today:

☐ ☐ ☐
☐ ☐ ☐ } _____ oz.

	Calories	Fat grams	Carbs/gms	Fiber/gms	Protein/gms	
DINNER Amount						
Time: [ ] Dinner Totals >						
SNACK Amount						
Time: [ ] Snack Totals >						

Do the math:

TODAY'S ~GRAND TOTALS~

Calories	Fat
Carbs	Fiber
Protein	
	#Fruit/Veg.

VITAMINS / SUPPLEMENTS / MEDS.

Description	AM Qty. PM

PHYSICAL ACTIVITY

Activity	Hrs./Min.	Qty.	Intensity Low Med. High	Cal/Bn

NOTES:

MET TODAY'S GOALS?

| 0% | 25% | 50% | 75% | 100% |

Day #						Weight:			

Day of the Week & Date   *Time*

FOOD OR BEVERAGE		Calories	Fat grams	Carbs/gms	Fiber/gms	Protein/gms		
BREAKFAST	Amount							
Time: Breakfast Totals >								
SNACK	Amount							
Time: Snack Totals >								
LUNCH	Amount							
Time: Lunch Totals >								
SNACK	Amount							
Time: Snack Totals >								
PAGE SUBTOTALS:								

8 oz. glasses of water consumed today:

☐ ☐ ☐ ☐
☐ ☐ ☐ } _____ oz.

		Calories	Fat grams	Carbs/gms	Fiber/gms	Protein/gms	
DINNER	Amount						
Time: Dinner Totals >							
SNACK	Amount						
Time: Snack Totals >							

Do the math:

TODAY'S ~GRAND TOTALS~

Calories

Fat

Carbs

Fiber

Protein

#Fruit/Veg.

VITAMINS / SUPPLEMENTS / MEDS.

Description	AM	Qty.	PM

PHYSICAL ACTIVITY

Activity	Hrs./Min.	Qty.	Intensity Low	Med.	High	Cal/Bn

NOTES:

MET TODAY'S GOALS?

0%　　25%　　50%　　75%　　100%

FOOD OR BEVERAGE	Amount	Calories	Fat grams	Carbs/gms	Fiber/gms	Protein/gms		
BREAKFAST	Amount							
Time: Breakfast Totals >								
SNACK	Amount							
Time: Snack Totals >								
LUNCH	Amount							
Time: Lunch Totals >								
SNACK	Amount							
Time: Snack Totals >								
PAGE SUBTOTALS:								

8 oz. glasses of water
consumed today:

☐ ☐ ☐ ☐
☐ ☐ ☐ } _____ oz.

	Amount	Calories	Fat grams	Carbs/gms	Fiber/gms	Protein/gms	
DINNER							
Time: ☐ Dinner Totals >							
SNACK	Amount						
Time: ☐ Snack Totals >							

Do the math:

TODAY'S ~GRAND TOTALS~

Calories	Fat
Carbs	Fiber
Protein	
	#Fruit/Veg.

VITAMINS/SUPPLEMENTS/MEDS.

Description	AM Qty. PM

PHYSICAL ACTIVITY

Activity	Hrs./Min.	Qty.	Intensity			Cal/Bn
			Low	Med.	High	

NOTES:

MET TODAY'S GOALS?

0%   25%   50%   75%   100%

Day #						Weight:		Time

Day of the Week & Date

FOOD OR BEVERAGE		Calories	Fat grams	Carbs/gms	Fiber/gms	Protein/gms	
BREAKFAST	Amount						
Time: Breakfast Totals >							
SNACK	Amount						
Time: Snack Totals >							
LUNCH	Amount						
Time: Lunch Totals >							
SNACK	Amount						
Time: Snack Totals >							
PAGE SUBTOTALS:							

8 oz. glasses of water
consumed today:

☐ ☐ ☐
☐ ☐ ☐ } _____ oz.

		Calories	Fat grams	Carbs/gms	Fiber/gms	Protein/gms	
DINNER	Amount						
Time:	Dinner Totals >						
SNACK	Amount						
Time:	Snack Totals >						

Do the math:

TODAY'S ~GRAND TOTALS~

Calories ☐   Fat ☐

Carbs ☐   Fiber ☐

Protein ☐   _____ ☐

_____ ☐   #Fruit/Veg. ☐

VITAMINS / SUPPLEMENTS / MEDS.

Description	AM Qty. PM

PHYSICAL ACTIVITY

Activity	Hrs./Min.	Qty.	Intensity Low | Med. | High	Cal/Bn

NOTES:

MET TODAY'S GOALS?

0%	25%	50%	75%	100%

Day #		Weight:	
			Time
	Day of the Week & Date		

FOOD OR BEVERAGE		Calories	Fat grams	Carbs/gms	Fiber/gms	Protein/gms	
BREAKFAST	Amount						
Time: Breakfast Totals >							
SNACK	Amount						
Time: Snack Totals >							
LUNCH	Amount						
Time: Lunch Totals >							
SNACK	Amount						
Time: Snack Totals >							
PAGE SUBTOTALS:							

8 oz. glasses of water
consummed today:

☐ ☐ ☐ ☐ } _____ oz.

		Calories	Fat grams	Carbs/gms	Fiber/gms	Protein/gms	

DINNER	Amount						

Time: [   ] Dinner Totals >

SNACK	Amount						

Time: [   ] Snack Totals >

Do the math:

TODAY'S ~GRAND TOTALS~

Calories	Fat
Carbs	Fiber
Protein	
	#Fruit/Veg.

VITAMINS / SUPPLEMENTS / MEDS.

Description	AM Qty. PM

PHYSICAL ACTIVITY

Activity	Hrs./Min.	Qty.	Intensity			Cal/Bn
			Low	Med.	High	

NOTES:

MET TODAY'S GOALS?

0%   25%   50%   75%   100%

| Day # | | | | Weight: | | | | |
| | | | | | Time | | | |

_____
Day of the Week & Date

FOOD OR BEVERAGE		Calories	Fat grams	Carbs/gms	Fiber/gms	Protein/gms		
BREAKFAST	Amount							
Time: Breakfast Totals >								
SNACK	Amount							
Time: Snack Totals >								
LUNCH	Amount							
Time: Lunch Totals >								
SNACK	Amount							
Time: Snack Totals >								
PAGE SUBTOTALS:								

8 oz. glasses of water consumed today: ☐☐☐☐ ☐☐☐☐ } _____ oz.

	Amount	Calories	Fat grams	Carbs/gms	Fiber/gms	Protein/gms	
DINNER							
Time:	Dinner Totals >						
SNACK	Amount						
Time:	Snack Totals >						

Do the math:

TODAY'S ~GRAND TOTALS~

Calories

Fat

Carbs

Fiber

Protein

_____

_____ #Fruit/Veg.

VITAMINS / SUPPLEMENTS / MEDS.

Description	AM	Qty.	PM

PHYSICAL ACTIVITY

Activity	Hrs./Min.	Qty.	Intensity Low / Med. / High	Cal/Bn

NOTES:

MET TODAY'S GOALS?

0%   25%   50%   75%   100%

Day #								Weight:	
									Time

Day of the Week & Date

FOOD OR BEVERAGE		Calories	Fat grams	Carbs/gms	Fiber/gms	Protein/gms	
BREAKFAST	Amount						
Time: Breakfast Totals >							
SNACK	Amount						
Time: Snack Totals >							
LUNCH	Amount						
Time: Lunch Totals >							
SNACK	Amount						
Time: Snack Totals >							
PAGE SUBTOTALS:							

8 oz. glasses of water consumed today:

☐ ☐ ☐ ☐
☐ ☐ ☐ ☐ } _____ oz.

		Calories	Fat grams	Carbs/gms	Fiber/gms	Protein/gms	
DINNER	Amount						
Time: ☐ Dinner Totals >							
SNACK	Amount						
Time: ☐ Snack Totals >							

Do the math:

TODAY'S ~GRAND TOTALS~

Calories	Fat
Carbs	Fiber
Protein	
	#Fruit/Veg.

VITAMINS/SUPPLEMENTS/MEDS.

Description	AM	Qty.	PM

PHYSICAL ACTIVITY

Activity	Hrs./Min.	Qty.	Intensity Low	Med.	High	Cal/Bn

NOTES:

MET TODAY'S GOALS?

| 0% | 25% | 50% | 75% | 100% |

MemoryMinder Journals, Inc.©

Day #								Weight:	

Day of the Week & Date

Time

FOOD OR BEVERAGE	Calories	Fat grams	Carbs/gms	Fiber/gms	Protein/gms	
BREAKFAST Amount						
Time: Breakfast Totals >						
SNACK Amount						
Time: Snack Totals >						
LUNCH Amount						
Time: Lunch Totals >						
SNACK Amount						
Time: Snack Totals >						
PAGE SUBTOTALS:						

8 oz. glasses of water consumed today:

☐ ☐ ☐ ☐
☐ ☐ ☐ ☐ } _____ oz.

		Calories	Fat grams	Carbs/gms	Fiber/gms	Protein/gms	
DINNER	Amount						
Time: ☐ Dinner Totals >							
SNACK	Amount						
Time: ☐ Snack Totals >							

Do the math:

TODAY'S ~GRAND TOTALS~

Calories	Fat
Carbs	Fiber
Protein	
	#Fruit/Veg.

VITAMINS / SUPPLEMENTS / MEDS.

Description	AM Qty. PM

PHYSICAL ACTIVITY

Activity	Hrs./Min.	Qty.	Intensity Low | Med. | High	Cal/Bn

NOTES:

MET TODAY'S GOALS?

0%	25%	50%	75%	100%

Day #			Weight:				

Day of the Week & Date

Time

FOOD OR BEVERAGE		Calories	Fat grams	Carbs/gms	Fiber/gms	Protein/gms	
BREAKFAST	Amount						
Time: Breakfast Totals >							
SNACK	Amount						
Time: Snack Totals >							
LUNCH	Amount						
Time: Lunch Totals >							
SNACK	Amount						
Time: Snack Totals >							
PAGE SUBTOTALS:							

8 oz. glasses of water consumed today:

☐ ☐ ☐ ☐
☐ ☐ ☐ } _____ oz.

	Amount	Calories	Fat grams	Carbs/gms	Fiber/gms	Protein/gms	
DINNER							
Time: ___ Dinner Totals >							
SNACK	Amount						
Time: ___ Snack Totals >							

Do the math:

TODAY'S ~GRAND TOTALS~

Calories	Fat
Carbs	Fiber
Protein	
	#Fruit/Veg.

VITAMINS / SUPPLEMENTS / MEDS.

Description	AM Qty. PM

PHYSICAL ACTIVITY

Activity	Hrs./Min.	Qty.	Intensity Low / Med. / High	Cal/Bn

NOTES:

MET TODAY'S GOALS?

0%   25%   50%   75%   100%

Weight:

Time

_____
Day of the Week & Date

FOOD OR BEVERAGE	Calories	Fat grams	Carbs/gms	Fiber/gms	Protein/gms	
BREAKFAST Amount						
Time: Breakfast Totals >						
SNACK Amount						
Time: Snack Totals >						
LUNCH Amount						
Time: Lunch Totals >						
SNACK Amount						
Time: Snack Totals >						
PAGE SUBTOTALS:						

8 oz. glasses of water
consumed today:

☐ ☐ ☐ ☐
☐ ☐ ☐ ☐ } _____ oz.

		Calories	Fat grams	Carbs/gms	Fiber/gms	Protein/gms	
DINNER	Amount						
Time:	Dinner Totals >						
SNACK	Amount						
Time:	Snack Totals >						

Do the math:

TODAY'S ~GRAND TOTALS~

Calories   Fat

Carbs   Fiber

Protein

_____

_____   #Fruit/Veg.

VITAMINS / SUPPLEMENTS / MEDS.

Description	AM Qty. PM

PHYSICAL ACTIVITY

Activity	Hrs./Min.	Qty.	Intensity Low / Med. / High	Cal/Bn

NOTES:

MET TODAY'S GOALS?

| 0% | 25% | 50% | 75% | 100% |

Weight:

Time

Day of the Week & Date

FOOD OR BEVERAGE	Calories	Fat grams	Carbs/gms	Fiber/gms	Protein/gms		
BREAKFAST Amount							
Time: Breakfast Totals >							
SNACK Amount							
Time: Snack Totals >							
LUNCH Amount							
Time: Lunch Totals >							
SNACK Amount							
Time: Snack Totals >							
PAGE SUBTOTALS:							

8 oz. glasses of water
consumed today:

☐ ☐ ☐ ☐
☐ ☐ ☐ } _____ oz.

		Calories	Fat grams	Carbs/gms	Fiber/gms	Protein/gms	
DINNER	Amount						
Time: Dinner Totals >							
SNACK	Amount						
Time; Snack Totals >							

Do the math:

TODAY'S ~GRAND TOTALS~

Calories	Fat
Carbs	Fiber
Protein	
	#Fruit/Veg.

VITAMINS / SUPPLEMENTS / MEDS.

Description	AM Qty. PM

PHYSICAL ACTIVITY

Activity	Hrs./Min.	Qty.	Intensity			Cal/Bn
			Low	Med.	High	

NOTES:

MET TODAY'S GOALS?

0%	25%	50%	75%	100%

| Day # | | | | | Weight: | | Time |

Day of the Week & Date

FOOD OR BEVERAGE	Calories	Fat grams	Carbs/gms	Fiber/gms	Protein/gms	
BREAKFAST Amount						
Time: Breakfast Totals >						
SNACK Amount						
Time: Snack Totals >						
LUNCH Amount						
Time: Lunch Totals >						
SNACK Amount						
Time: Snack Totals >						
PAGE SUBTOTALS:						

MemoryMinder Journals, Inc.©

8 oz. glasses of water
consumed today:

☐ ☐ ☐ } _____ oz.
☐ ☐ ☐

		Calories	Fat grams	Carbs/gms	Fiber/gms	Protein/gms	
DINNER	Amount						
Time: Dinner Totals >							
SNACK	Amount						
Time: Snack Totals >							

Do the math:

TODAY'S ~GRAND TOTALS~

Calories	Fat
Carbs	Fiber
Protein	
	#Fruit/Veg.

VITAMINS / SUPPLEMENTS / MEDS.

Description	AM Qty. PM

PHYSICAL ACTIVITY

Activity	Hrs./Min.	Qty.	Intensity Low Med. High	Cal/Bn

NOTES:

MET TODAY'S GOALS?

0%   25%   50%   75%   100%

MemoryMinder Journals, Inc. ©

Day #		Weight:					
	Day of the Week & Date						*Time*

FOOD OR BEVERAGE	Calories	Fat grams	Carbs/gms	Fiber/gms	Protein/gms		
BREAKFAST Amount							
Time: Breakfast Totals >							
SNACK Amount							
Time: Snack Totals >							
LUNCH Amount							
Time: Lunch Totals >							
SNACK Amount							
Time: Snack Totals >							
PAGE SUBTOTALS:							

8 oz. glasses of water
consumed today:

⬜⬜⬜⬜ } _____ oz.
⬜⬜⬜⬜

	Calories	Fat grams	Carbs/gms	Fiber/gms	Protein/gms	
DINNER Amount						
Time: [ ] Dinner Totals >						
SNACK Amount						
Time: [ ] Snack Totals >						

Do the math:

TODAY'S ~GRAND TOTALS~

Calories	Fat
Carbs	Fiber
Protein	
	#Fruit/Veg.

VITAMINS / SUPPLEMENTS / MEDS.

Description	AM	Qty.	PM

PHYSICAL ACTIVITY

Activity	Hrs./Min.	Qty.	Intensity			Cal/Bn
			Low	Med.	High	

NOTES:

MET TODAY'S GOALS?

| 0% | 25% | 50% | 75% | 100% |

Day #			Weight:	
	Day of the Week & Date			*Time*

FOOD OR BEVERAGE	Calories	Fat grams	Carbs/gms	Fiber/gms	Protein/gms	
BREAKFAST Amount						
Time: Breakfast Totals >						
SNACK Amount						
Time: Snack Totals >						
LUNCH Amount						
Time: Lunch Totals >						
SNACK Amount						
Time: Snack Totals >						
PAGE SUBTOTALS:						

8 oz. glasses of water
consumed today:

☐ ☐ ☐ ☐
☐ ☐ ☐ ☐ } _____ oz.

		Calories	Fat grams	Carbs/gms	Fiber/gms	Protein/gms	
DINNER	Amount						
Time: Dinner Totals >							
SNACK	Amount						
Time: Snack Totals >							

Do the math:

TODAY'S ~GRAND TOTALS~

Calories	Fat
Carbs	Fiber
Protein	
	#Fruit/Veg.

VITAMINS / SUPPLEMENTS / MEDS.

Description	AM	Qty.	PM

PHYSICAL ACTIVITY

Activity	Hrs./Min.	Qty.	Intensity			Cal/Bn
			Low	Med.	High	

NOTES:

MET TODAY'S GOALS?

0%   25%   50%   75%   100%

MemoryMinder Journals, Inc.©

Day #						Weight:			Time

Day of the Week & Date

FOOD OR BEVERAGE		Calories	Fat grams	Carbs/gms	Fiber/gms	Protein/gms		
BREAKFAST	Amount							
Time: Breakfast Totals >								
SNACK	Amount							
Time: Snack Totals >								
LUNCH	Amount							
Time: Lunch Totals >								
SNACK	Amount							
Time: Snack Totals >								
PAGE SUBTOTALS:								

8 oz. glasses of water
consumed today:

☐ ☐ ☐ } _____ oz.
☐ ☐ ☐

		Calories	Fat grams	Carbs/gms	Fiber/gms	Protein/gms	
DINNER	Amount						
Time: Dinner Totals >							
SNACK	Amount						
Time: Snack Totals >							

Do the math:

TODAY'S ~GRAND TOTALS~

Calories	Fat
Carbs	Fiber
Protein	_____
_____	#Fruit/Veg.

VITAMINS / SUPPLEMENTS / MEDS.

Description	AM	Qty.	PM

PHYSICAL ACTIVITY

Activity	Hrs./Min.	Qty.	Intensity			Cal/Bn
			Low	Med.	High	

NOTES:

MET TODAY'S GOALS?

0%	25%	50%	75%	100%

Day #		Weight:	
	Day of the Week & Date		*Time*

FOOD OR BEVERAGE		Calories	Fat grams	Carbs/gms	Fiber/gms	Protein/gms	
BREAKFAST	Amount						
Time: Breakfast Totals >							
SNACK	Amount						
Time: Snack Totals >							
LUNCH	Amount						
Time: Lunch Totals >							
SNACK	Amount						
Time: Snack Totals >							
PAGE SUBTOTALS:							

8 oz. glasses of water
consumed today:

☐☐☐☐ }
☐☐☐☐ _____ oz.

	Calories	Fat grams	Carbs/gms	Fiber/gms	Protein/gms	
DINNER Amount						
Time: Dinner Totals >						
SNACK Amount						
Time: Snack Totals >						

Do the math:

TODAY'S ~GRAND TOTALS~

Calories   Fat

Carbs   Fiber

Protein

_____   #Fruit/Veg.

VITAMINS / SUPPLEMENTS / MEDS.

Description	AM Qty. PM

PHYSICAL ACTIVITY

Activity	Hrs./Min.	Qty.	Intensity			Cal/Bn
			Low	Med.	High	

NOTES:

MET TODAY'S GOALS?

0%	25%	50%	75%	100%

MemoryMinder Journals, Inc.©

Day #					Weight:		

Day of the Week & Date

Time

FOOD OR BEVERAGE	Calories	Fat grams	Carbs/gms	Fiber/gms	Protein/gms		
BREAKFAST Amount							
Time: Breakfast Totals >							
SNACK Amount							
Time: Snack Totals >							
LUNCH Amount							
Time: Lunch Totals >							
SNACK Amount							
Time: Snack Totals >							
PAGE SUBTOTALS:							

8 oz. glasses of water consumed today:

} _____ oz.

	Calories	Fat grams	Carbs/gms	Fiber/gms	Protein/gms	
DINNER Amount						
Time: Dinner Totals >						
SNACK Amount						
Time: Snack Totals >						

Do the math:

TODAY'S ~GRAND TOTALS~

Calories

Fat

Carbs

Fiber

Protein

_____

_____

#Fruit/Veg.

VITAMINS / SUPPLEMENTS / MEDS.

Description	AM	Qty.	PM

PHYSICAL ACTIVITY

Activity	Hrs./Min.	Qty.	Intensity			Cal/Bn
			Low	Med.	High	

NOTES:

MET TODAY'S GOALS?

0%	25%	50%	75%	100%

Weight:

Time

Day of the Week & Date

FOOD OR BEVERAGE

		Calories	Fat grams	Carbs/gms	Fiber/gms	Protein/gms	
BREAKFAST	Amount						
Time: Breakfast Totals >							
SNACK	Amount						
Time: Snack Totals >							
LUNCH	Amount						
Time: Lunch Totals >							
SNACK	Amount						
Time: Snack Totals >							
PAGE SUBTOTALS:							

8 oz. glasses of water
consumed today:

☐ ☐ ☐
☐ ☐ ☐ } _____ oz.

		Calories	Fat grams	Carbs/gms	Fiber/gms	Protein/gms	
DINNER	Amount						
Time:	Dinner Totals >						
SNACK	Amount						
Time:	Snack Totals >						

Do the math:

TODAY'S ~GRAND TOTALS~

Calories	Fat
Carbs	Fiber
Protein	
	#Fruit/Veg.

VITAMINS / SUPPLEMENTS / MEDS.

Description	AM	Qty.	PM

PHYSICAL ACTIVITY

Activity	Hrs./Min.	Qty.	Intensity Low / Med. / High	Cal/Bn

NOTES:

MET TODAY'S GOALS?

0% 25% 50% 75% 100%

Day #								Weight:	Time

Day of the Week & Date

FOOD OR BEVERAGE		Calories	Fat grams	Carbs/gms	Fiber/gms	Protein/gms		
BREAKFAST	Amount							
Time: Breakfast Totals >								
SNACK	Amount							
Time: Snack Totals >								
LUNCH	Amount							
Time: Lunch Totals >								
SNACK	Amount							
Time: Snack Totals >								
PAGE SUBTOTALS:								

8 oz. glasses of water
consumed today:

☐ ☐ ☐ ☐
☐ ☐ ☐ ☐ } _____ oz.

	Calories	Fat grams	Carbs/gms	Fiber/gms	Protein/gms	
DINNER Amount						
Time: Dinner Totals >						
SNACK Amount						
Time; Snack Totals >						

Do the math:

TODAY'S ~GRAND TOTALS~

Calories	Fat
Carbs	Fiber
Protein	
	#Fruit/Veg.

VITAMINS / SUPPLEMENTS / MEDS.

Description	AM	Qty.	PM

PHYSICAL ACTIVITY

Activity	Hrs./Min.	Qty.	Intensity (Low / Med. / High)	Cal/Bn

NOTES:

MET TODAY'S GOALS?

0%   25%   50%   75%   100%

Day #						Weight:	
							Time

Day of the Week & Date

FOOD OR BEVERAGE		Calories	Fat grams	Carbs/gms	Fiber/gms	Protein/gms	
BREAKFAST	Amount						
Time: Breakfast Totals >							
SNACK	Amount						
Time: Snack Totals >							
LUNCH	Amount						
Time: Lunch Totals >							
SNACK	Amount						
Time: Snack Totals >							
PAGE SUBTOTALS:							

8 oz. glasses of water
consumed today:

☐ ☐ ☐ ☐
☐ ☐ ☐ ☐ } _____ oz.

		Calories	Fat grams	Carbs/gms	Fiber/gms	Protein/gms	
DINNER	Amount						
Time: Dinner Totals >							
SNACK	Amount						
Time: Snack Totals >							

Do the math:

TODAY'S ~GRAND TOTALS~

Calories

Fat

Carbs

Fiber

Protein

_____

_____

#Fruit/Veg.

VITAMINS / SUPPLEMENTS / MEDS.

Description	AM	Qty.	PM

PHYSICAL ACTIVITY

Activity	Hrs./Min.	Qty.	Intensity			Cal/Bn
			Low	Med.	High	

NOTES:

MET TODAY'S GOALS?

0%　　　25%　　　50%　　　75%　　　100%

_____

Day of the Week & Date

FOOD OR BEVERAGE		Calories	Fat grams	Carbs/gms	Fiber/gms	Protein/gms	
BREAKFAST	Amount						
Time: Breakfast Totals >							
SNACK	Amount						
Time: Snack Totals >							
LUNCH	Amount						
Time: Lunch Totals >							
SNACK	Amount						
Time: Snack Totals >							
PAGE SUBTOTALS:							

8 oz. glasses of water
consumed today:

☐☐☐☐ ⎫
☐☐☐☐ ⎬ _____ oz.

		Calories	Fat grams	Carbs/gms	Fiber/gms	Protein/gms	
DINNER	Amount						
Time:	Dinner Totals >						
SNACK	Amount						
Time:	Snack Totals >						

Do the math:

TODAY'S ~GRAND TOTALS~

Calories   Fat

Carbs   Fiber

Protein

_____   #Fruit/Veg.

VITAMINS / SUPPLEMENTS / MEDS.

Description	AM	Qty.	PM

PHYSICAL ACTIVITY

Activity	Hrs./Min.	Qty.	Intensity			Cal/Bn
			Low	Med.	High	

NOTES:

MET TODAY'S GOALS?

0%   25%   50%   75%   100%

Day #				Weight:			Time

Day of the Week & Date

FOOD OR BEVERAGE		Calories	Fat grams	Carbs/gms	Fiber/gms	Protein/gms	
BREAKFAST	Amount						
Time: Breakfast Totals >							
SNACK	Amount						
Time: Snack Totals >							
LUNCH	Amount						
Time: Lunch Totals >							
SNACK	Amount						
Time: Snack Totals >							
PAGE SUBTOTALS:							

8 oz. glasses of water consumed today:

☐☐☐☐
☐☐☐☐ } _____ oz.

	Amount	Calories	Fat grams	Carbs/gms	Fiber/gms	Protein/gms	
DINNER							
Time:	Dinner Totals >						
SNACK	Amount						
Time:	Snack Totals >						

Do the math:

TODAY'S ~GRAND TOTALS~

Calories	Fat
Carbs	Fiber
Protein	_____
_____	#Fruit/Veg.

VITAMINS / SUPPLEMENTS / MEDS.

Description	AM Qty. PM

PHYSICAL ACTIVITY

Activity	Hrs./Min.	Qty.	Intensity Low Med. High	Cal/Bn

NOTES:

MET TODAY'S GOALS?

0%   25%   50%   75%   100%

FOOD OR BEVERAGE		Calories	Fat grams	Carbs/gms	Fiber/gms	Protein/gms	
BREAKFAST	Amount						
Time: Breakfast Totals >							
SNACK	Amount						
Time: Snack Totals >							
LUNCH	Amount						
Time: Lunch Totals >							
SNACK	Amount						
Time: Snack Totals >							
PAGE SUBTOTALS:							

8 oz. glasses of water consumed today:

☐ ☐ ☐ ☐
☐ ☐ ☐ ☐ } _____ oz.

		Calories	Fat grams	Carbs/gms	Fiber/gms	Protein/gms	
DINNER	Amount						
Time:	Dinner Totals >						
SNACK	Amount						
Time:	Snack Totals >						

Do the math:

TODAY'S ~GRAND TOTALS~

Calories	Fat
Carbs	Fiber
Protein	
	#Fruit/Veg.

VITAMINS / SUPPLEMENTS / MEDS.

Description	AM	Qty. PM

PHYSICAL ACTIVITY

Activity	Hrs./Min.	Qty.	Intensity			Cal/Bn
			Low	Med.	High	

NOTES:

MET TODAY'S GOALS?

0% — 25% — 50% — 75% — 100%

MemoryMinder Journals, Inc.©

Day #		Weight:					

Day of the Week & Date

Time

FOOD OR BEVERAGE		Calories	Fat grams	Carbs/gms	Fiber/gms	Protein/gms	
BREAKFAST	Amount						
Time: Breakfast Totals >							
SNACK	Amount						
Time: Snack Totals >							
LUNCH	Amount						
Time: Lunch Totals >							
SNACK	Amount						
Time: Snack Totals >							
PAGE SUBTOTALS:							

8 oz. glasses of water
consumed today:

☐ ☐ ☐ ☐ } _____ oz.
☐ ☐ ☐ ☐

	Amount	Calories	Fat grams	Carbs/gms	Fiber/gms	Protein/gms	
DINNER							
Time: Dinner Totals >							
SNACK	Amount						
Time: Snack Totals >							

Do the math:

TODAY'S ~GRAND TOTALS~

Calories		Fat	
Carbs		Fiber	
Protein			
		#Fruit/Veg.	

VITAMINS / SUPPLEMENTS / MEDS.

Description	AM	Qty.	PM

PHYSICAL ACTIVITY

Activity	Hrs./Min.	Qty.	Intensity (Low / Med. / High)	Cal/Bn

NOTES:

MET TODAY'S GOALS?

0%   25%   50%   75%   100%

Day #				Weight:			

Day of the Week & Date

Time

FOOD OR BEVERAGE	Calories	Fat grams	Carbs/gms	Fiber/gms	Protein/gms		
BREAKFAST Amount							
Time: Breakfast Totals >							
SNACK Amount							
Time: Snack Totals >							
LUNCH Amount							
Time: Lunch Totals >							
SNACK Amount							
Time: Snack Totals >							
PAGE SUBTOTALS:							

8 oz. glasses of water
consumed today:

☐ ☐ ☐ ☐ } _____ oz.
☐ ☐ ☐ ☐

	Calories	Fat grams	Carbs/gms	Fiber/gms	Protein/gms	
DINNER Amount						
Time: Dinner Totals >						
SNACK Amount						
Time: Snack Totals >						

Do the math:

TODAY'S ~GRAND TOTALS~

Calories	Fat
Carbs	Fiber
Protein	
	#Fruit/Veg.

VITAMINS / SUPPLEMENTS / MEDS.

Description	AM Qty. PM

PHYSICAL ACTIVITY

Activity	Hrs./Min.	Qty.	Intensity (Low / Med. / High)	Cal/Bn

NOTES:

MET TODAY'S GOALS?

0%   25%   50%   75%   100%

Day #			Weight:			Time

Day of the Week & Date

FOOD OR BEVERAGE		Calories	Fat grams	Carbs/gms	Fiber/gms	Protein/gms	
BREAKFAST	Amount						
Time: Breakfast Totals >							
SNACK	Amount						
Time: Snack Totals >							
LUNCH	Amount						
Time: Lunch Totals >							
SNACK	Amount						
Time: Snack Totals >							
PAGE SUBTOTALS:							

8 oz. glasses of water
consumed today:

☐ ☐ ☐ ☐
☐ ☐ ☐ ☐ } _____ oz.

	Calories	Fat grams	Carbs/gms	Fiber/gms	Protein/gms	
DINNER Amount						
Time: Dinner Totals >						
SNACK Amount						
Time: Snack Totals >						

Do the math:

TODAY'S ~GRAND TOTALS~

Calories ☐   Fat ☐

Carbs ☐   Fiber ☐

Protein ☐   ☐

☐   #Fruit/Veg. ☐

VITAMINS / SUPPLEMENTS / MEDS.

Description	AM Qty. PM

PHYSICAL ACTIVITY

Activity	Hrs./Min.	Qty.	Intensity Low / Med. / High	Cal/Bn

NOTES:

MET TODAY'S GOALS?

0%   25%   50%   75%   100%

Day #			Weight:			Time

Day of the Week & Date

FOOD OR BEVERAGE		Calories	Fat grams	Carbs/gms	Fiber/gms	Protein/gms	
BREAKFAST	Amount						
Time: Breakfast Totals >							
SNACK	Amount						
Time: Snack Totals >							
LUNCH	Amount						
Time: Lunch Totals >							
SNACK	Amount						
Time: Snack Totals >							
PAGE SUBTOTALS:							

8 oz. glasses of water
consumed today:

☐ ☐ ☐ ☐
☐ ☐ ☐ ☐ } _____ oz.

		Calories	Fat grams	Carbs/gms	Fiber/gms	Protein/gms	
DINNER	Amount						
Time:	Dinner Totals >						
SNACK	Amount						
Time:	Snack Totals >						

Do the math:

TODAY'S
~GRAND TOTALS~

Calories   Fat

Carbs   Fiber

Protein

_____   #Fruit/Veg.

VITAMINS / SUPPLEMENTS / MEDS.

Description	AM Qty. PM

PHYSICAL ACTIVITY

Activity	Hrs./Min.	Qty.	Intensity Low Med. High	Cal/Bn

NOTES:

MET TODAY'S GOALS?

0%   25%   50%   75%   100%

Day #								Weight:	

Time

Day of the Week & Date

FOOD OR BEVERAGE		Calories	Fat grams	Carbs/gms	Fiber/gms	Protein/gms	
BREAKFAST	Amount						
Time: Breakfast Totals >							
SNACK	Amount						
Time: Snack Totals >							
LUNCH	Amount						
Time: Lunch Totals >							
SNACK	Amount						
Time: Snack Totals >							
PAGE SUBTOTALS:							

8 oz. glasses of water consumed today:

☐ ☐ ☐
☐ ☐ ☐ } _____ oz.

	Amount	Calories	Fat grams	Carbs/gms	Fiber/gms	Protein/gms	
DINNER							
Time: Dinner Totals >							
SNACK Amount							
Time: Snack Totals >							

Do the math:

TODAY'S ~GRAND TOTALS~

Calories	Fat
Carbs	Fiber
Protein	
	#Fruit/Veg.

VITAMINS / SUPPLEMENTS / MEDS.

Description	AM	Qty.	PM

PHYSICAL ACTIVITY

Activity	Hrs./Min.	Qty.	Intensity Low / Med. / High	Cal/Bn

NOTES:

MET TODAY'S GOALS?

0%   25%   50%   75%   100%

Day #								Weight:	

Day of the Week & Date

Time

FOOD OR BEVERAGE		Calories	Fat grams	Carbs/gms	Fiber/gms	Protein/gms	
BREAKFAST	Amount						
Time: Breakfast Totals >							
SNACK	Amount						
Time: Snack Totals >							
LUNCH	Amount						
Time: Lunch Totals >							
SNACK	Amount						
Time: Snack Totals >							
PAGE SUBTOTALS:							

8 oz. glasses of water
consumed today:

☐ ☐ ☐ ☐
☐ ☐ ☐ ☐ } _____ oz.

	Amount	Calories	Fat grams	Carbs/gms	Fiber/gms	Protein/gms	
DINNER							
Time:	Dinner Totals >						
SNACK	Amount						
Time:	Snack Totals >						

Do the math:

TODAY'S ~GRAND TOTALS~

Calories	Fat
Carbs	Fiber
Protein	
_____	_____ #Fruit/Veg.

VITAMINS / SUPPLEMENTS / MEDS.

Description	AM	Qty.	PM

PHYSICAL ACTIVITY

Activity	Hrs./Min.	Qty.	Intensity			Cal/Bn
			Low	Med.	High	

NOTES:

MET TODAY'S GOALS?

0%	25%	50%	75%	100%

Day #			Weight:				Time	

Day of the Week & Date

FOOD OR BEVERAGE		Calories	Fat grams	Carbs/gms	Fiber/gms	Protein/gms		
BREAKFAST	Amount							
Time: Breakfast Totals >								
SNACK	Amount							
Time: Snack Totals >								
LUNCH	Amount							
Time: Lunch Totals >								
SNACK	Amount							
Time: Snack Totals >								
PAGE SUBTOTALS:								

8 oz. glasses of water
consumed today:

☐ ☐ ☐ ☐ } _____ oz.
☐ ☐ ☐ ☐

	Amount	Calories	Fat grams	Carbs/gms	Fiber/gms	Protein/gms	
DINNER							
Time: Dinner Totals >							
SNACK Amount							
Time: Snack Totals >							

Do the math:

TODAY'S ~GRAND TOTALS~

Calories	Fat
Carbs	Fiber
Protein	_____
_____	#Fruit/Veg.

VITAMINS / SUPPLEMENTS / MEDS.

Description	AM Qty. PM

PHYSICAL ACTIVITY

Activity	Hrs./Min.	Qty.	Intensity (Low / Med. / High)	Cal/Bn

NOTES:

MET TODAY'S GOALS?

0%   25%   50%   75%   100%

Day #						Weight:		Time

Day of the Week & Date

FOOD OR BEVERAGE		Calories	Fat grams	Carbs/gms	Fiber/gms	Protein/gms		
BREAKFAST	Amount							
Time: Breakfast Totals >								
SNACK	Amount							
Time: Snack Totals >								
LUNCH	Amount							
Time: Lunch Totals >								
SNACK	Amount							
Time: Snack Totals >								
PAGE SUBTOTALS:								

8 oz. glasses of water consumed today:

☐ ☐ ☐ ☐
☐ ☐ ☐ ☐ } _____ oz.

	Amount	Calories	Fat grams	Carbs/gms	Fiber/gms	Protein/gms	
DINNER							
Time: Dinner Totals >							
SNACK Amount							
Time: Snack Totals >							

Do the math:

TODAY'S ~GRAND TOTALS~

Calories	Fat
Carbs	Fiber
Protein	
	#Fruit/Veg.

VITAMINS / SUPPLEMENTS / MEDS.

Description	AM	Qty.	PM

PHYSICAL ACTIVITY

Activity	Hrs./Min.	Qty.	Intensity Low Med. High	Cal/Bn

NOTES:

MET TODAY'S GOALS?

0%   25%   50%   75%   100%

Day #						

Day of the Week & Date

Weight: _Time_

FOOD OR BEVERAGE		Calories	Fat grams	Carbs/gms	Fiber/gms	Protein/gms	
BREAKFAST	Amount						
Time: Breakfast Totals >							
SNACK	Amount						
Time: Snack Totals >							
LUNCH	Amount						
Time: Lunch Totals >							
SNACK	Amount						
Time: Snack Totals >							
PAGE SUBTOTALS:							

8 oz. glasses of water
consumed today:

☐ ☐ ☐ ☐ } _____ oz.
☐ ☐ ☐ ☐

	Amount	Calories	Fat grams	Carbs/gms	Fiber/gms	Protein/gms	
DINNER							
Time: [ ] Dinner Totals >							
SNACK	Amount						
Time: [ ] Snack Totals >							

Do the math:

TODAY'S ~GRAND TOTALS~

Calories	Fat
Carbs	Fiber
Protein	
	#Fruit/Veg.

VITAMINS / SUPPLEMENTS / MEDS.

Description	AM	Qty. PM

PHYSICAL ACTIVITY

Activity	Hrs./Min.	Qty.	Intensity Low / Med. / High	Cal/Bn

NOTES:

MET TODAY'S GOALS?

| 0% | 25% | 50% | 75% | 100% |

Weight:

Time

Day of the Week & Date

FOOD OR BEVERAGE

		Calories	Fat grams	Carbs/gms	Fiber/gms	Protein/gms	
BREAKFAST	Amount						
Time: Breakfast Totals >							
SNACK	Amount						
Time: Snack Totals >							
LUNCH	Amount						
Time: Lunch Totals >							
SNACK	Amount						
Time: Snack Totals >							
PAGE SUBTOTALS:							

8 oz. glasses of water
consumed today:

☐ ☐ ☐ ☐ }
☐ ☐ ☐ ☐ } _____ oz.

		Calories	Fat grams	Carbs/gms	Fiber/gms	Protein/gms	
DINNER	Amount						
Time: Dinner Totals >							
SNACK	Amount						
Time: Snack Totals >							

Do the math:

TODAY'S ~GRAND TOTALS~

Calories	Fat
Carbs	Fiber
Protein	
	#Fruit/Veg.

VITAMINS / SUPPLEMENTS / MEDS.

Description	AM Qty. PM

PHYSICAL ACTIVITY

Activity	Hrs./Min.	Qty.	Intensity			Cal/Bn
			Low	Med.	High	

NOTES:

MET TODAY'S GOALS?

| 0% | 25% | 50% | 75% | 100% |

Day #								Weight:	Time

Day of the Week & Date

FOOD OR BEVERAGE		Calories	Fat grams	Carbs/gms	Fiber/gms	Protein/gms	
BREAKFAST	Amount						
Time: Breakfast Totals >							
SNACK	Amount						
Time: Snack Totals >							
LUNCH	Amount						
Time: Lunch Totals >							
SNACK	Amount						
Time: Snack Totals >							
PAGE SUBTOTALS:							

8 oz. glasses of water consumed today:

☐ ☐ ☐ ☐
☐ ☐ ☐ ☐ } _____ oz.

		Calories	Fat grams	Carbs/gms	Fiber/gms	Protein/gms	
DINNER	Amount						
Time: Dinner Totals >							
SNACK	Amount						
Time: Snack Totals >							

Do the math:

TODAY'S ~GRAND TOTALS~

Calories   Fat

Carbs   Fiber

Protein

_____

_____   #Fruit/Veg.

VITAMINS / SUPPLEMENTS / MEDS.

Description	AM	Qty.	PM

PHYSICAL ACTIVITY

Activity	Hrs./Min.	Qty.	Intensity Low / Med. / High	Cal/Bn

NOTES:

MET TODAY'S GOALS?

0% 25% 50% 75% 100%

Day #			Weight:				

Day of the Week & Date

Time

FOOD OR BEVERAGE	Calories	Fat grams	Carbs/gms	Fiber/gms	Protein/gms		
BREAKFAST Amount							
Time: Breakfast Totals >							
SNACK Amount							
Time: Snack Totals >							
LUNCH Amount							
Time: Lunch Totals >							
SNACK Amount							
Time: Snack Totals >							
PAGE SUBTOTALS:							

8 oz. glasses of water consumed today:

☐ ☐ ☐ ☐
☐ ☐ ☐ } _____ oz.

	Calories	Fat grams	Carbs/gms	Fiber/gms	Protein/gms	
DINNER Amount						
Time: Dinner Totals >						
SNACK Amount						
Time: Snack Totals >						

Do the math:

TODAY'S ~GRAND TOTALS~

Calories	Fat
Carbs	Fiber
Protein	
_____	_____ #Fruit/Veg.

VITAMINS / SUPPLEMENTS / MEDS.

Description	AM	Qty. PM

PHYSICAL ACTIVITY

Activity	Hrs./Min.	Qty.	Intensity Low | Med. | High	Cal/Bn

NOTES:

MET TODAY'S GOALS?

0%   25%   50%   75%   100%

Day #			Weight:		
				Time	

Day of the Week & Date

FOOD OR BEVERAGE		Calories	Fat grams	Carbs/gms	Fiber/gms	Protein/gms	
BREAKFAST	Amount						
Time: Breakfast Totals >							
SNACK	Amount						
Time: Snack Totals >							
LUNCH	Amount						
Time: Lunch Totals >							
SNACK	Amount						
Time: Snack Totals >							
PAGE SUBTOTALS:							

8 oz. glasses of water
consumed today:

☐ ☐ ☐ ☐
☐ ☐ ☐ ☐ } _____ oz.

		Calories	Fat grams	Carbs/gms	Fiber/gms	Protein/gms	
DINNER	Amount						
Time: Dinner Totals >							
SNACK	Amount						
Time: Snack Totals >							

Do the math:

TODAY'S ~GRAND TOTALS~

Calories

Fat

Carbs

Fiber

Protein

_____

_____

#Fruit/Veg.

VITAMINS / SUPPLEMENTS / MEDS.

Description	AM Qty. PM

PHYSICAL ACTIVITY

Activity	Hrs./Min.	Qty.	Intensity Low | Med. | High	Cal/Bn

NOTES:

MET TODAY'S GOALS?

0%   25%   50%   75%   100%

MemoryMinder Journals, Inc.©

Day #		Weight:		
	Day of the Week & Date		Time	

FOOD OR BEVERAGE		Calories	Fat grams	Carbs/gms	Fiber/gms	Protein/gms	
BREAKFAST	Amount						
Time: Breakfast Totals >							
SNACK	Amount						
Time: Snack Totals >							
LUNCH	Amount						
Time: Lunch Totals >							
SNACK	Amount						
Time: Snack Totals >							
PAGE SUBTOTALS:							

8 oz. glasses of water
consumed today:

☐☐☐☐
☐☐☐☐ } _____ oz.

	Amount	Calories	Fat grams	Carbs/gms	Fiber/gms	Protein/gms	
DINNER							
Time: Dinner Totals >							
SNACK	Amount						
Time: Snack Totals >							

Do the math:

TODAY'S ~GRAND TOTALS~

Calories

Fat

Carbs

Fiber

Protein

#Fruit/Veg.

VITAMINS / SUPPLEMENTS / MEDS.

Description	AM	Qty.	PM

PHYSICAL ACTIVITY

Activity	Hrs./Min.	Qty.	Intensity Low / Med. / High	Cal/Bn

NOTES:

MET TODAY'S GOALS?

0%   25%   50%   75%   100%

Day #			Weight:	Time

Day of the Week & Date

FOOD OR BEVERAGE		Calories	Fat grams	Carbs/gms	Fiber/gms	Protein/gms	
BREAKFAST	Amount						
Time: Breakfast Totals >							
SNACK	Amount						
Time: Snack Totals >							
LUNCH	Amount						
Time: Lunch Totals >							
SNACK	Amount						
Time: Snack Totals >							
PAGE SUBTOTALS:							

8 oz. glasses of water consumed today:

☐ ☐ ☐ ☐
☐ ☐ ☐ ☐ } _____ oz.

		Calories	Fat grams	Carbs/gms	Fiber/gms	Protein/gms	
DINNER	Amount						
Time:	Dinner Totals >						
SNACK	Amount						
Time:	Snack Totals >						

Do the math:

TODAY'S ~GRAND TOTALS~

Calories

Fat

Carbs

Fiber

Protein

_____

_____ #Fruit/Veg.

VITAMINS / SUPPLEMENTS / MEDS.

Description	AM	Qty.	PM

PHYSICAL ACTIVITY

Activity	Hrs./Min.	Qty.	Intensity Low / Med. / High	Cal/Bn

NOTES:

MET TODAY'S GOALS?

0%	25%	50%	75%	100%

Day #								Weight:	Time

Day of the Week & Date

FOOD OR BEVERAGE		Calories	Fat grams	Carbs/gms	Fiber/gms	Protein/gms		
BREAKFAST	Amount							
Time: Breakfast Totals >								
SNACK	Amount							
Time: Snack Totals >								
LUNCH	Amount							
Time: Lunch Totals >								
SNACK	Amount							
Time: Snack Totals >								
PAGE SUBTOTALS:								

8 oz. glasses of water consumed today:

☐☐☐☐
☐☐☐☐ } _____ oz.

| Calories | Fat grams | Carbs/gms | Fiber/gms | Protein/gms |

DINNER	Amount						

Time: Dinner Totals >

SNACK	Amount						

Time: Snack Totals >

Do the math:

TODAY'S ~GRAND TOTALS~

Calories

Fat

Carbs

Fiber

Protein

_____

_____

#Fruit/Veg.

VITAMINS / SUPPLEMENTS / MEDS.

Description	AM	Qty.	PM

PHYSICAL ACTIVITY

Activity	Hrs./Min.	Qty.	Intensity			Cal/Bn
			Low	Med.	High	

NOTES:

MET TODAY'S GOALS?

| 0% | 25% | 50% | 75% | 100% |

Day #				Weight:	
	Day of the Week & Date			Time	

FOOD OR BEVERAGE		Calories	Fat grams	Carbs/gms	Fiber/gms	Protein/gms	
BREAKFAST	Amount						
Time: Breakfast Totals >							
SNACK	Amount						
Time: Snack Totals >							
LUNCH	Amount						
Time: Lunch Totals >							
SNACK	Amount						
Time: Snack Totals >							
PAGE SUBTOTALS:							

8 oz. glasses of water consumed today:

☐☐☐☐
☐☐☐☐ } _____ oz.

	Amount	Calories	Fat grams	Carbs/gms	Fiber/gms	Protein/gms	
DINNER							
Time: Dinner Totals >							
SNACK	Amount						
Time: Snack Totals >							

Do the math:

TODAY'S ~GRAND TOTALS~

Calories

Fat

Carbs

Fiber

Protein

_____

_____   #Fruit/Veg.

VITAMINS / SUPPLEMENTS / MEDS.

Description	AM	Qty.	PM

PHYSICAL ACTIVITY

Activity	Hrs./Min.	Qty.	Intensity			Cal/Bn
			Low	Med.	High	

NOTES:

MET TODAY'S GOALS?

0%   25%   50%   75%   100%

Day #								Weight:		
									Time	

Day of the Week & Date

FOOD OR BEVERAGE		Calories	Fat grams	Carbs/gms	Fiber/gms	Protein/gms		
BREAKFAST	Amount							
Time: Breakfast Totals >								
SNACK	Amount							
Time: Snack Totals >								
LUNCH	Amount							
Time: Lunch Totals >								
SNACK	Amount							
Time: Snack Totals >								
PAGE SUBTOTALS:								

8 oz. glasses of water
consumed today:

☐ ☐ ☐ ☐
☐ ☐ ☐ ☐ } _____ oz.

	Calories	Fat grams	Carbs/gms	Fiber/gms	Protein/gms	
DINNER Amount						
Time: Dinner Totals >						
SNACK Amount						
Time: Snack Totals >						

Do the math:

TODAY'S
~GRAND TOTALS~

Calories	Fat
Carbs	Fiber
Protein	_____
_____	#Fruit/Veg.

VITAMINS / SUPPLEMENTS / MEDS.

Description	AM Qty. PM

PHYSICAL ACTIVITY

Activity	Hrs./Min.	Qty.	Intensity Low / Med. / High	Cal/Bn

NOTES:

MET TODAY'S GOALS?

0%   25%   50%   75%   100%

MemoryMinder Journals, Inc.©

Day #								Weight:	
		Day of the Week & Date						Time	

FOOD OR BEVERAGE		Calories	Fat grams	Carbs/gms	Fiber/gms	Protein/gms	
BREAKFAST	Amount						
Time:	Breakfast Totals >						
SNACK	Amount						
Time:	Snack Totals >						
LUNCH	Amount						
Time:	Lunch Totals >						
SNACK	Amount						
Time:	Snack Totals >						
PAGE SUBTOTALS:							

8 oz. glasses of water
consumed today:

☐ ☐ ☐ } _____ oz.
☐ ☐ ☐

	Calories	Fat grams	Carbs/gms	Fiber/gms	Protein/gms	
DINNER Amount						
Time: Dinner Totals >						
SNACK Amount						
Time: Snack Totals >						

Do the math:

TODAY'S ~GRAND TOTALS~

Calories

Fat

Carbs

Fiber

Protein

_____

_____   #Fruit/Veg.

VITAMINS / SUPPLEMENTS / MEDS.

Description	AM	Qty.	PM

PHYSICAL ACTIVITY

Activity	Hrs./Min.	Qty.	Intensity			Cal/Bn
			Low	Med.	High	

NOTES:

MET TODAY'S GOALS?

0%	25%	50%	75%	100%

Day #			Weight:		
				Time	

Day of the Week & Date

FOOD OR BEVERAGE		Calories	Fat grams	Carbs/gms	Fiber/gms	Protein/gms	
BREAKFAST	Amount						
Time: Breakfast Totals >							
SNACK	Amount						
Time: Snack Totals >							
LUNCH	Amount						
Time: Lunch Totals >							
SNACK	Amount						
Time: Snack Totals >							
PAGE SUBTOTALS:							

8 oz. glasses of water
consumed today:

☐ ☐ ☐ ☐ }
☐ ☐ ☐ ☐ _____ oz.

DINNER	Amount	Calories	Fat grams	Carbs/gms	Fiber/gms	Protein/gms	
Time: Dinner Totals >							

SNACK	Amount						
Time: Snack Totals >							

Do the math:

TODAY'S ~GRAND TOTALS~

Calories	Fat
Carbs	Fiber
Protein	
	#Fruit/Veg.

VITAMINS / SUPPLEMENTS / MEDS.		
Description	AM	Qty. PM

PHYSICAL ACTIVITY					
Activity	Hrs./Min.	Qty.	Intensity Low Med. High		Cal/Bn

NOTES:

MET TODAY'S GOALS?

0%	25%	50%	75%	100%

Day #			Weight:			Time	

Day of the Week & Date

FOOD OR BEVERAGE		Calories	Fat grams	Carbs/gms	Fiber/gms	Protein/gms	
BREAKFAST	Amount						
Time: Breakfast Totals >							
SNACK	Amount						
Time: Snack Totals >							
LUNCH	Amount						
Time: Lunch Totals >							
SNACK	Amount						
Time: Snack Totals >							
PAGE SUBTOTALS:							

8 oz. glasses of water consumed today:

} _____ oz.

		Calories	Fat grams	Carbs/gms	Fiber/gms	Protein/gms	
DINNER	Amount						
Time: Dinner Totals >							
SNACK	Amount						
Time: Snack Totals >							

Do the math:

TODAY'S ~GRAND TOTALS~

Calories

Fat

Carbs

Fiber

Protein

_____

_____   #Fruit/Veg.

VITAMINS / SUPPLEMENTS / MEDS.

Description	AM	Qty.	PM

PHYSICAL ACTIVITY

Activity	Hrs./Min.	Qty.	Intensity Low / Med. / High	Cal/Bn

NOTES:

MET TODAY'S GOALS?

0%   25%   50%   75%   100%

Day #		Weight:	
			Time
	Day of the Week & Date		

FOOD OR BEVERAGE	Calories	Fat grams	Carbs/gms	Fiber/gms	Protein/gms	
BREAKFAST Amount						
Time: Breakfast Totals >						
SNACK Amount						
Time: Snack Totals >						
LUNCH Amount						
Time: Lunch Totals >						
SNACK Amount						
Time: Snack Totals >						
PAGE SUBTOTALS:						

8 oz. glasses of water
consumed today:

☐ ☐ ☐ ☐ }
☐ ☐ ☐ ☐ _____oz.

		Calories	Fat grams	Carbs/gms	Fiber/gms	Protein/gms	
DINNER	Amount						
Time: Dinner Totals >							
SNACK	Amount						
Time: Snack Totals >							

Do the math:

TODAY'S ~GRAND TOTALS~

Calories ☐ Fat ☐

Carbs ☐ Fiber ☐

Protein ☐ ☐

☐ #Fruit/Veg. ☐

VITAMINS / SUPPLEMENTS / MEDS.

Description	AM Qty. PM

PHYSICAL ACTIVITY

Activity	Hrs./Min.	Qty.	Intensity Low Med. High	Cal/Bn

NOTES:

MET TODAY'S GOALS?

0%   25%   50%   75%   100%

Day #		Weight:				Time	

Day of the Week & Date

FOOD OR BEVERAGE		Calories	Fat grams	Carbs/gms	Fiber/gms	Protein/gms	
BREAKFAST	Amount						
Time: Breakfast Totals >							
SNACK	Amount						
Time: Snack Totals >							
LUNCH	Amount						
Time: Lunch Totals >							
SNACK	Amount						
Time: Snack Totals >							
PAGE SUBTOTALS:							

8 oz. glasses of water
consumed today:

☐ ☐ ☐ ☐ } _____ oz.
☐ ☐ ☐ ☐

DINNER	Amount	Calories	Fat grams	Carbs/gms	Fiber/gms	Protein/gms	
Time:	Dinner Totals >						
SNACK	Amount						
Time:	Snack Totals >						

Do the math:

TODAY'S ~GRAND TOTALS~

Calories	Fat
Carbs	Fiber
Protein	
	#Fruit/Veg.

VITAMINS / SUPPLEMENTS / MEDS.			
Description	AM	Qty.	PM

PHYSICAL ACTIVITY

Activity	Hrs./Min.	Qty.	Intensity			Cal/Bn
			Low	Med.	High	

NOTES:

MET TODAY'S GOALS?

0% 25% 50% 75% 100%

Day #		Day of the Week & Date	Weight:			Time	

FOOD OR BEVERAGE		Calories	Fat grams	Carbs/gms	Fiber/gms	Protein/gms	
BREAKFAST	Amount						
Time: Breakfast Totals >							
SNACK	Amount						
Time: Snack Totals >							
LUNCH	Amount						
Time: Lunch Totals >							
SNACK	Amount						
Time: Snack Totals >							
PAGE SUBTOTALS:							

8 oz. glasses of water consumed today:

☐ ☐ ☐ ☐
☐ ☐ ☐ ☐ } _____ oz.

	Calories	Fat grams	Carbs/gms	Fiber/gms	Protein/gms	
DINNER Amount						
Time: Dinner Totals >						
SNACK Amount						
Time. Snack Totals >						

Do the math:

TODAY'S ~GRAND TOTALS~

Calories	Fat
Carbs	Fiber
Protein	
	#Fruit/Veg.

VITAMINS / SUPPLEMENTS / MEDS.

Description	AM	Qty. PM

PHYSICAL ACTIVITY

Activity	Hrs./Min.	Qty.	Intensity Low / Med. / High	Cal/Bn

NOTES:

MET TODAY'S GOALS?

0% 25% 50% 75% 100%

Day #							Weight:	

Day of the Week & Date

Time

FOOD OR BEVERAGE		Calories	Fat grams	Carbs/gms	Fiber/gms	Protein/gms	
BREAKFAST	Amount						
Time: Breakfast Totals >							
SNACK	Amount						
Time: Snack Totals >							
LUNCH	Amount						
Time: Lunch Totals >							
SNACK	Amount						
Time: Snack Totals >							
PAGE SUBTOTALS:							

8 oz. glasses of water consumed today:

☐ ☐ ☐
☐ ☐ ☐ } _____ oz.

	Amount	Calories	Fat grams	Carbs/gms	Fiber/gms	Protein/gms		
DINNER								
Time:	Dinner Totals >							
SNACK	Amount							
Time:	Snack Totals >							

Do the math:

TODAY'S ~GRAND TOTALS~

Calories

Fat

Carbs

Fiber

Protein

#Fruit/Veg.

VITAMINS / SUPPLEMENTS / MEDS.

Description	AM	Qty.	PM

PHYSICAL ACTIVITY

Activity	Hrs./Min.	Qty.	Intensity Low	Med.	High	Cal/Bn

NOTES:

MET TODAY'S GOALS?

| 0% | 25% | 50% | 75% | 100% |

Day #			Weight:					Time	

Day of the Week & Date

FOOD OR BEVERAGE		Calories	Fat grams	Carbs/gms	Fiber/gms	Protein/gms		
BREAKFAST	Amount							
Time: Breakfast Totals >								
SNACK	Amount							
Time: Snack Totals >								
LUNCH	Amount							
Time: Lunch Totals >								
SNACK	Amount							
Time: Snack Totals >								
PAGE SUBTOTALS:								

8 oz. glasses of water
consumed today:

☐ ☐ ☐ ☐
☐ ☐ ☐ ☐ } _____ oz.

	Calories	Fat grams	Carbs/gms	Fiber/gms	Protein/gms	
DINNER　　Amount						
Time: ☐　Dinner Totals >						
SNACK　　Amount						
Time: ☐　Snack Totals >						

Do the math:

TODAY'S ~GRAND TOTALS~

Calories	Fat
Carbs	Fiber
Protein	
	#Fruit/Veg.

VITAMINS / SUPPLEMENTS / MEDS.

Description	AM Qty. PM

PHYSICAL ACTIVITY

Activity	Hrs./Min.	Qty.	Intensity Low　Med.　High	Cal/Bn

NOTES:

MET TODAY'S GOALS?

0%　　25%　　50%　　75%　　100%

Day #							Weight:		

Day of the Week & Date

Time

FOOD OR BEVERAGE		Calories	Fat grams	Carbs/gms	Fiber/gms	Protein/gms	
BREAKFAST	Amount						
Time: Breakfast Totals >							
SNACK	Amount						
Time: Snack Totals >							
LUNCH	Amount						
Time: Lunch Totals >							
SNACK	Amount						
Time: Snack Totals >							
PAGE SUBTOTALS:							

8 oz. glasses of water consumed today:

☐ ☐ ☐
☐ ☐ ☐ } _____ oz.

		Calories	Fat grams	Carbs/gms	Fiber/gms	Protein/gms	
DINNER	Amount						
Time: Dinner Totals >							
SNACK	Amount						
Time: Snack Totals >							

Do the math:

TODAY'S ~GRAND TOTALS~

Calories | Fat

Carbs | Fiber

Protein |

_____ | #Fruit/Veg.

VITAMINS / SUPPLEMENTS / MEDS.

Description	AM	Qty.	PM

PHYSICAL ACTIVITY

Activity	Hrs./Min.	Qty.	Intensity (Low / Med. / High)	Cal/Bn

NOTES:

MET TODAY'S GOALS?

0% 25% 50% 75% 100%

MemoryMinder Journals, Inc.©

MemoryMinder Journals, Inc.©

Day #		Weight:	
	Day of the Week & Date		Time

FOOD OR BEVERAGE		Calories	Fat grams	Carbs/gms	Fiber/gms	Protein/gms	
BREAKFAST	Amount						
Time: Breakfast Totals >							
SNACK	Amount						
Time: Snack Totals >							
LUNCH	Amount						
Time: Lunch Totals >							
SNACK	Amount						
Time: Snack Totals >							
PAGE SUBTOTALS:							

8 oz. glasses of water
consumed today:

☐☐☐☐
☐☐☐☐ } _____ oz.

		Calories	Fat grams	Carbs/gms	Fiber/gms	Protein/gms	
DINNER	Amount						
Time: Dinner Totals >							
SNACK	Amount						
Time: Snack Totals >							

Do the math:

TODAY'S ~GRAND TOTALS~

Calories	Fat
Carbs	Fiber
Protein	_____
_____	#Fruit/Veg.

VITAMINS / SUPPLEMENTS / MEDS.

Description	AM Qty. PM

PHYSICAL ACTIVITY

Activity	Hrs./Min.	Qty.	Intensity			Cal/Bn
			Low	Med.	High	

NOTES:

MET TODAY'S GOALS?

0%	25%	50%	75%	100%

Day #		
	Day of the Week & Date	Weight: _Time_

FOOD OR BEVERAGE	Calories	Fat grams	Carbs/gms	Fiber/gms	Protein/gms	
BREAKFAST Amount						
Time: Breakfast Totals >						
SNACK Amount						
Time: Snack Totals >						
LUNCH Amount						
Time: Lunch Totals >						
SNACK Amount						
Time: Snack Totals >						
PAGE SUBTOTALS:						

8 oz. glasses of water
consumed today:

☐ ☐ ☐ ☐
☐ ☐ ☐ } _____ oz.

	Amount	Calories	Fat grams	Carbs/gms	Fiber/gms	Protein/gms	
DINNER	Amount						
Time: Dinner Totals >							
SNACK	Amount						
Time: Snack Totals >							

Do the math:

**TODAY'S
~GRAND TOTALS~**

Calories | Fat

Carbs | Fiber

Protein

_____

_____ #Fruit/Veg

VITAMINS / SUPPLEMENTS / MEDS.

Description	AM	Qty.	PM

PHYSICAL ACTIVITY

Activity	Hrs./Min.	Qty.	Intensity Low / Med. / High	Cal/Bn

NOTES:

MET TODAY'S GOALS?

| 0% | 25% | 50% | 75% | 100% |

Day #							Weight:		

Day of the Week & Date

Time

FOOD OR BEVERAGE		Calories	Fat grams	Carbs/gms	Fiber/gms	Protein/gms		
BREAKFAST	Amount							
Time: Breakfast Totals >								
SNACK	Amount							
Time: Snack Totals >								
LUNCH	Amount							
Time: Lunch Totals >								
SNACK	Amount							
Time: Snack Totals >								
PAGE SUBTOTALS:								

MemoryMinder Journals, Inc.©

8 oz. glasses of water
consumed today:

☐ ☐ ☐ ☐ }
☐ ☐ ☐ ☐ _____ oz.

		Calories	Fat grams	Carbs/gms	Fiber/gms	Protein/gms	
DINNER	Amount						
Time: Dinner Totals >							
SNACK	Amount						
Time: Snack Totals >							

Do the math:

TODAY'S ~GRAND TOTALS~

Calories	Fat
Carbs	Fiber
Protein	
	#Fruit/Veg.

VITAMINS / SUPPLEMENTS / MEDS.

Description	AM Qty. PM

PHYSICAL ACTIVITY

Activity	Hrs./Min.	Qty.	Intensity			Cal/Bn
			Low	Med.	High	

NOTES:

MET TODAY'S GOALS?

0%	25%	50%	75%	100%

Day #		Weight:		
			Time	

Day of the Week & Date

FOOD OR BEVERAGE		Calories	Fat grams	Carbs/gms	Fiber/gms	Protein/gms		
BREAKFAST	Amount							
Time: Breakfast Totals >								
SNACK	Amount							
Time: Snack Totals >								
LUNCH	Amount							
Time: Lunch Totals >								
SNACK	Amount							
Time: Snack Totals >								
PAGE SUBTOTALS:								

8 oz. glasses of water consumed today:

☐ ☐ ☐ ☐
☐ ☐ ☐ ☐ } _____oz.

	Calories	Fat grams	Carbs/gms	Fiber/gms	Protein/gms	
DINNER Amount						
Time: Dinner Totals >						
SNACK Amount						
Time: Snack Totals >						

Do the math:

TODAY'S ~GRAND TOTALS~

Calories

Fat

Carbs

Fiber

Protein

_____

_____

#Fruit/Veg.

VITAMINS/SUPPLEMENTS/MEDS.

Description	AM	Qty.	PM

PHYSICAL ACTIVITY

Activity	Hrs./Min.	Qty.	Intensity Low	Med.	High	Cal/Bn

NOTES:

MET TODAY'S GOALS?

0%   25%   50%   75%   100%

Day #			Weight:	
				Time

Day of the Week & Date

FOOD OR BEVERAGE		Calories	Fat grams	Carbs/gms	Fiber/gms	Protein/gms		
BREAKFAST	Amount							
Time: Breakfast Totals >								
SNACK	Amount							
Time: Snack Totals >								
LUNCH	Amount							
Time: Lunch Totals >								
SNACK	Amount							
Time: Snack Totals >								
PAGE SUBTOTALS:								

8 oz. glasses of water
consumed today:

☐ ☐ ☐ ☐ } _____ oz.
☐ ☐ ☐ ☐

		Calories	Fat grams	Carbs/gms	Fiber/gms	Protein/gms	
DINNER	Amount						
Time:	Dinner Totals >						
SNACK	Amount						
Time:	Snack Totals >						

Do the math:

TODAY'S ~GRAND TOTALS~

Calories	Fat
Carbs	Fiber
Protein	
	#Fruit/Veg.

VITAMINS / SUPPLEMENTS / MEDS.

Description	AM	Qty.	PM

PHYSICAL ACTIVITY

Activity	Hrs./Min.	Qty.	Intensity			Cal/Bn
			Low	Med.	High	

NOTES:

MET TODAY'S GOALS?

0%   25%   50%   75%   100%

Day #						Weight:		

Day of the Week & Date

Time

FOOD OR BEVERAGE		Calories	Fat grams	Carbs/gms	Fiber/gms	Protein/gms	
BREAKFAST	Amount						
Time: Breakfast Totals >							
SNACK	Amount						
Time: Snack Totals >							
LUNCH	Amount						
Time: Lunch Totals >							
SNACK	Amount						
Time: Snack Totals >							
PAGE SUBTOTALS:							

8 oz. glasses of water
consumed today:

☐☐☐☐ }
☐☐☐☐ _____ oz.

		Calories	Fat grams	Carbs/gms	Fiber/gms	Protein/gms	
DINNER	Amount						
Time:	Dinner Totals >						
SNACK	Amount						
Time:	Snack Totals >						

Do the math:

TODAY'S ~GRAND TOTALS~

Calories Fat

Carbs Fiber

Protein

#Fruit/Veg.

VITAMINS / SUPPLEMENTS / MEDS.

Description	AM	Qty.	PM

PHYSICAL ACTIVITY

Activity	Hrs./Min.	Qty.	Intensity Low / Med. / High	Cal/Bn

NOTES:

MET TODAY'S GOALS?

0%   25%   50%   75%   100%

Day #						Weight:	
							Time

Day of the Week & Date

FOOD OR BEVERAGE		Calories	Fat grams	Carbs/gms	Fiber/gms	Protein/gms	
BREAKFAST	Amount						
Time: Breakfast Totals >							
SNACK	Amount						
Time: Snack Totals >							
LUNCH	Amount						
Time: Lunch Totals >							
SNACK	Amount						
Time: Snack Totals >							
PAGE SUBTOTALS:							

8 oz. glasses of water
consumed today:

☐ ☐ ☐ ☐
☐ ☐ ☐ ☐ } _____ oz.

	Calories	Fat grams	Carbs/gms	Fiber/gms	Protein/gms	
DINNER Amount						
Time: Dinner Totals >						
SNACK Amount						
Time: Snack Totals >						

Do the math:

TODAY'S ~GRAND TOTALS~

Calories   Fat

Carbs   Fiber

Protein

_____   #Fruit/Veg.

VITAMINS / SUPPLEMENTS / MEDS.

Description	AM Qty. PM

PHYSICAL ACTIVITY

Activity	Hrs./Min.	Qty.	Intensity Low | Med. | High	Cal/Bn

NOTES:

MET TODAY'S GOALS?

0%   25%   50%   75%   100%

MemoryMinder Journals, Inc ©

Day of the Week & Date

FOOD OR BEVERAGE

	Calories	Fat grams	Carbs/gms	Fiber/gms	Protein/gms		
BREAKFAST Amount							
Time: Breakfast Totals >							
SNACK Amount							
Time: Snack Totals >							
LUNCH Amount							
Time: Lunch Totals >							
SNACK Amount							
Time: Snack Totals >							
PAGE SUBTOTALS:							

8 oz. glasses of water consumed today:

☐ ☐ ☐ ☐
☐ ☐ ☐ ☐ } _____ oz.

		Calories	Fat grams	Carbs/gms	Fiber/gms	Protein/gms	
DINNER	Amount						
Time:	Dinner Totals >						
SNACK	Amount						
Time:	Snack Totals >						

Do the math:

TODAY'S ~GRAND TOTALS~

Calories	Fat
Carbs	Fiber
Protein	
	#Fruit/Veg.

VITAMINS / SUPPLEMENTS / MEDS.

Description	AM Qty. PM

PHYSICAL ACTIVITY

Activity	Hrs./Min.	Qty.	Intensity			Cal/Bn
			Low	Med.	High	

NOTES:

MET TODAY'S GOALS?

0%	25%	50%	75%	100%

Day #				Weight:		Time

Day of the Week & Date

FOOD OR BEVERAGE		Calories	Fat grams	Carbs/gms	Fiber/gms	Protein/gms	
BREAKFAST	Amount						
Time: Breakfast Totals >							
SNACK	Amount						
Time: Snack Totals >							
LUNCH	Amount						
Time: Lunch Totals >							
SNACK	Amount						
Time: Snack Totals >							
PAGE SUBTOTALS:							

8 oz. glasses of water consumed today:

☐ ☐ ☐ ☐ } _____ oz.
☐ ☐ ☐ ☐

		Calories	Fat grams	Carbs/gms	Fiber/gms	Protein/gms		
DINNER	Amount							
Time:	Dinner Totals >							
SNACK	Amount							
Time:	Snack Totals >							

Do the math:

TODAY'S ~GRAND TOTALS~

Calories

Fat

Carbs

Fiber

Protein

_____

_____

#Fruit/Veg.

VITAMINS / SUPPLEMENTS / MEDS.

Description	AM	Qty.	PM

PHYSICAL ACTIVITY

Activity	Hrs./Min.	Qty.	Intensity			Cal/Bn
			Low	Med.	High	

NOTES:

MET TODAY'S GOALS?

| 0% | 25% | 50% | 75% | 100% |

Day #			Weight:					

Day of the Week & Date

Time

FOOD OR BEVERAGE	Calories	Fat grams	Carbs/gms	Fiber/gms	Protein/gms	
BREAKFAST Amount						
Time: Breakfast Totals >						
SNACK Amount						
Time: Snack Totals >						
LUNCH Amount						
Time: Lunch Totals >						
SNACK Amount						
Time: Snack Totals >						
PAGE SUBTOTALS:						

8 oz. glasses of water
consumed today:

□□□□
□□□□ } _____ oz.

	Calories	Fat grams	Carbs/gms	Fiber/gms	Protein/gms	
DINNER Amount						
Time: Dinner Totals >						
SNACK Amount						
Time: Snack Totals >						

Do the math:

TODAY'S ~GRAND TOTALS~

Calories   Fat

Carbs   Fiber

Protein

_____   _____ #Fruit/Veg.

VITAMINS / SUPPLEMENTS / MEDS.
Description   AM Qty. PM

PHYSICAL ACTIVITY

Activity	Hrs./Min.	Qty.	Intensity Low	Med.	High	Cal/Bn

NOTES:

MET TODAY'S GOALS?

0%   25%   50%   75%   100%

Day #							Weight:	Time

Day of the Week & Date

FOOD OR BEVERAGE		Calories	Fat grams	Carbs/gms	Fiber/gms	Protein/gms	
BREAKFAST	Amount						
Time: Breakfast Totals >							
SNACK	Amount						
Time: Snack Totals >							
LUNCH	Amount						
Time: Lunch Totals >							
SNACK	Amount						
Time: Snack Totals >							
PAGE SUBTOTALS:							

8 oz. glasses of water
consumed today:

☐ ☐ ☐ ☐ }
☐ ☐ ☐ ☐ _____ oz.

		Calories	Fat grams	Carbs/gms	Fiber/gms	Protein/gms	
DINNER	Amount						
Time:	Dinner Totals >						
SNACK	Amount						
Time:	Snack Totals >						

Do the math:

TODAY'S ~GRAND TOTALS~

Calories

Fat

Carbs

Fiber

Protein

#Fruit/Veg.

VITAMINS / SUPPLEMENTS / MEDS.

Description	AM	Qty.	PM

PHYSICAL ACTIVITY

Activity	Hrs./Min.	Qty.	Intensity			Cal/Bn
			Low	Med.	High	

NOTES:

MET TODAY'S GOALS?

0%　　　25%　　　50%　　　75%　　　100%

Day #					Weight:			Time

Day of the Week & Date

FOOD OR BEVERAGE		Calories	Fat grams	Carbs/gms	Fiber/gms	Protein/gms		
BREAKFAST	Amount							
Time: Breakfast Totals >								
SNACK	Amount							
Time: Snack Totals >								
LUNCH	Amount							
Time: Lunch Totals >								
SNACK	Amount							
Time: Snack Totals >								
PAGE SUBTOTALS:								

8 oz. glasses of water
consumed today:

☐ ☐ ☐ ☐
☐ ☐ ☐ ☐ } _____ oz.

	Amount	Calories	Fat grams	Carbs/gms	Fiber/gms	Protein/gms	
DINNER							
Time:	Dinner Totals >						
SNACK	Amount						
Time:	Snack Totals >						

Do the math:

TODAY'S ~GRAND TOTALS~

Calories

Fat

Carbs

Fiber

Protein

_____

_____

#Fruit/Veg.

VITAMINS / SUPPLEMENTS / MEDS.

Description	AM	Qty.	PM

PHYSICAL ACTIVITY

Activity	Hrs./Min.	Qty.	Intensity (Low / Med. / High)	Cal/Bn

NOTES:

MET TODAY'S GOALS?

0%   25%   50%   75%   100%

Day #		Weight:						Time	

Day of the Week & Date

FOOD OR BEVERAGE		Calories	Fat grams	Carbs/gms	Fiber/gms	Protein/gms		
BREAKFAST	Amount							
Time: Breakfast Totals >								
SNACK	Amount							
Time: Snack Totals >								
LUNCH	Amount							
Time: Lunch Totals >								
SNACK	Amount							
Time: Snack Totals >								
PAGE SUBTOTALS:								

8 oz. glasses of water consumed today:

⬜⬜⬜⬜
⬜⬜⬜⬜ } _____ oz.

	Calories	Fat grams	Carbs/gms	Fiber/gms	Protein/gms	
DINNER Amount						
Time: Dinner Totals >						
SNACK Amount						
Time: Snack Totals >						

Do the math:

TODAY'S ~GRAND TOTALS~

Calories   Fat

Carbs   Fiber

Protein   _____

_____   #Fruit/Veg.

VITAMINS / SUPPLEMENTS / MEDS.

Description	AM Qty. PM

PHYSICAL ACTIVITY

Activity	Hrs./Min.	Qty.	Intensity (Low / Med. / High)	Cal/Bn

NOTES:

MET TODAY'S GOALS?

0%   25%   50%   75%   100%

Day #						Weight:	Time

Day of the Week & Date

FOOD OR BEVERAGE		Calories	Fat grams	Carbs/gms	Fiber/gms	Protein/gms	
BREAKFAST	Amount						
Time: Breakfast Totals >							
SNACK	Amount						
Time: Snack Totals >							
LUNCH	Amount						
Time: Lunch Totals >							
SNACK	Amount						
Time: Snack Totals >							
PAGE SUBTOTALS:							

8 oz. glasses of water consumed today:

☐ ☐ ☐ ☐
☐ ☐ ☐ ☐ } _____ oz.

		Calories	Fat grams	Carbs/gms	Fiber/gms	Protein/gms	
DINNER	Amount						
Time:	Dinner Totals >						
SNACK	Amount						
Time:	Snack Totals >						

Do the math:

TODAY'S ~GRAND TOTALS~

Calories

Fat

Carbs

Fiber

Protein

_____

_____

#Fruit/Vcg.

VITAMINS / SUPPLEMENTS / MEDS.

Description	AM	Qty.	PM

PHYSICAL ACTIVITY

Activity	Hrs./Min.	Qty.	Intensity Low / Med. / High	Cal/Bn

NOTES:

MET TODAY'S GOALS?

0%   25%   50%   75%   100%

| Day # | | | | | | Weight: | | Time |

FOOD OR BEVERAGE	Calories	Fat grams	Carbs/gms	Fiber/gms	Protein/gms	
BREAKFAST Amount						
Time: Breakfast Totals >						
SNACK Amount						
Time: Snack Totals >						
LUNCH Amount						
Time: Lunch Totals >						
SNACK Amount						
Time: Snack Totals >						
PAGE SUBTOTALS:						

Day of the Week & Date

MemoryMinder Journals, Inc.©

8 oz. glasses of water consumed today:

☐☐☐☐ } _____ oz.
☐☐☐☐

		Calories	Fat grams	Carbs/gms	Fiber/gms	Protein/gms	
DINNER	Amount						
Time: Dinner Totals >							
SNACK	Amount						
Time: Snack Totals >							

Do the math:

MemoryMinder Journals, Inc.©

VITAMINS / SUPPLEMENTS / MEDS.

Description	AM	Qty. PM

TODAY'S ~GRAND TOTALS~

Calories	Fat
Carbs	Fiber
Protein	
	#Fruit/Veg.

PHYSICAL ACTIVITY

Activity	Hrs./Min.	Qty.	Intensity			Cal/Bn
			Low	Med.	High	

NOTES:

MET TODAY'S GOALS?

0%　　　25%　　　50%　　　75%　　　100%

MemoryMinder Journals, Inc.©

Day #						Weight:				Time

Day of the Week & Date

FOOD OR BEVERAGE		Calories	Fat grams	Carbs/gms	Fiber/gms	Protein/gms		
BREAKFAST	Amount							
Time: Breakfast Totals >								
SNACK	Amount							
Time: Snack Totals >								
LUNCH	Amount							
Time: Lunch Totals >								
SNACK	Amount							
Time: Snack Totals >								
PAGE SUBTOTALS:								

MemoryMinder Journals, Inc.©

8 oz. glasses of water consumed today:

☐ ☐ ☐ ☐ } _____ oz.
☐ ☐ ☐ ☐

		Calories	Fat grams	Carbs/gms	Fiber/gms	Protein/gms		
DINNER	Amount							
Time: Dinner Totals >								
SNACK	Amount							
Time: Snack Totals >								

Do the math:

TODAY'S ~GRAND TOTALS~

Calories | Fat

Carbs | Fiber

Protein | _____

_____ | #Fruit/Veg.

VITAMINS / SUPPLEMENTS / MEDS.

Description	AM	Qty.	PM

PHYSICAL ACTIVITY

Activity	Hrs./Min.	Qty.	Intensity Low	Med.	High	Cal/Bn

NOTES:

MET TODAY'S GOALS?

0% 25% 50% 75% 100%

Additional Records

- *Favorite Foods Facts*
- *Graph Records*
- *Weekly Progress Chart*
- *Reference Calendar*

Favorite Foods Facts*

Use these pages to look up common foods; add your favorites to personalize the list.

~FOOD OR BEVERAGE~	AMT.	Calories	Fat grams	Carbs/gms	Fiber/gms	Protein/gms		
A								
Almonds	1 oz	167	14.8	5.8	3.1	5.7		
Apple, medium	1	81	.5	21.1	3.7	.3		
Applesauce/sweetened	1/2 c.	97	.2	25.5	1.5	.2		
Applesauce/unsweetnd	1/2 c.	53	.1	13.8	1.5	.2		
Apricot, medium	3	51	.4	11.8	2.5	1.5		
Artichoke, medium	1	60	.2	13.4	6.5	4.2		
Avocado, medium	1	306	30.0	12.0	4.7	3.6		
B	AMT.							
Bacon, pan fried	2 slice	70	6.0	0	0	5.0		
Bagel (plain)	1	150	1.0	34.0	1.0	9.0		
Baked beans	1/2 c.	170	1.0	21.0	7.0	6.0		
Banana (medium)	1	105	.6	26.7	2.7	1.2		
Beef, ground, lean	4 oz.	308	20.9	0	0	28.0		
Beef, T-Bone, lean	4 oz.	243	11.8	0	0	31.9		
Beer, regular	12 oz.	146	0	13.2	.7	.9		
Blueberries, fresh	1/2 c.	41	.3	10.2	2.0	.5		
Bread, wheat	1 slice	70	1.0	12.0	1.4	3.0		
Broccoli, chopped	1/2 c.	12	.2	2.3	1.3	1.3		
Burger, *Big Mac*	1	560	31.0	45.0	3.0	26.0		
Burger, *BK Whopper*	1	640	39.0	45.0	3.0	27.0		
Butter	1 Tb.	100	11.4	0	0	.1		

*Food count listings are approximate and may vary slightly.

Favorite Foods Facts
continued

~FOOD OR BEVERAGE~	AMT.	Calories	Fat grams	Carbs/gms	Fiber/gms	Protein/gms		
C								
Candy:								
M&M's, plain	1/4 c.	210	9.0	30.0	1.0	2.0		
Jelly Belly jelly beans	35	140	0	37.0	0	0		
Cantalope, cubed	1/2 c.	29	.2	6.7	.6	.7		
Carrot, whole, 7.5"	1	31	.1	7.3	2.2	.7		
Cashews, roasted	18	163	8.1	13.7	1.1	4.6		
Celery, 7.5"stalk	1	6	.1	1.5	.7	.3		
Cheese, cheddar	1 oz.	110	9.0	1.0	0	7.0		
Chicken, light meat	4 oz.	196	5.1	0	0	35.1		
Chips, Potato, reg.	15	160	10.0	14.0	1.0	2.0		
Chips, *Ruffles*, lowfat	16	140	7.0	18.0	1.0	2.0		
Chips, *Pringles*-nofat	15	70	0	15.0	2.0	2.0		
Coffee, brewed	6 oz.	4	0	.8	0	.1		
Cookie, *Oreo*	3	160	7.0	23.0	1.0	1.0		
Corn, frozen	1/2c.	80	1.0	17.0	2.0	2.0		
Corn flakes	1 oz.	100	0	24.0	1.0	2.0		
Cottage cheese, lo-fat	1/2 c.	100	2.0	4.0	0	14.0		
Crackers, *Ritz*	5	80	4.0	10.0	0	1.0		
Cream, 25% fat	1 Tb.	37	3.8	.5	0	.4		

C

Favorite Foods Facts
continued

~FOOD OR BEVERAGE~	AMT.	Calories	Fat grams	Carbs/gms	Fiber/gms	Protein/gms		
D-E								
Dates, pitted	5	120	0	32.0	3.0	1.0		
Dill pickle, whole	1	13	0	2.7	0	.4		
Donut, glazed	1	250	12.0	33.0	1.4	3.0		
Egg:								
Raw, large, whole	1	75	5.0	.6	0	6.3		
Raw, white only	1	17	0	.3	0	3.5		
Hardboiled, chopped	1 c.	210	14.4	1.5	0	17.1		
F-G	AMT.							
Flatfish (sole, etc.)	4 oz.	104	1.4	0	0	21.4		
French fries, *McD's,*	1 sm bag	210	10.0	26.0	2.0	3.0		
Frankfurter, *O. Mayer*	1	150	13.0	1.0	0	5.0		
Frosting, canned/choc.	2 Tb.	130	5.0	22.0	0	.1		
Grapes, seedless	10	36	.3	8.9	.3	.3		
Grapejuice, purple, 100%	1/2 c.	80	0	20.0	0	0		
Grapefruit, pink, med.	1/2	46	.1	11.9	1.4	.6		
Green beans, boiled	1/2c.	22	.2	4.9	2.0	1.2		

D E F G

Favorite Foods Facts
continued

~FOOD OR BEVERAGE~	AMT.	Calories	Fat grams	Carbs/gms	Fiber/gms	Protein/gms.		
H-I								
Halibut, baked	4 oz.	159	3.3	0	0	30.3		
Ham, diced, lean	4 oz.	249	12.5	0	0	32.1		
Honey	1Tb.	60	0	16.0	0	0		
Hummus	2 Tb.	50	3.5	5.0	1.0	2.0		
Ice cream, Vanilla *Haagen Dazs*	1/2 c.	260	17.0	23.0	0	5.0		
Ice cream bar, *Dove*	12	80	19.0	23.0	1	5.0		
Ice milk, lo-fat	1/2 c.	100	2.0	17.0	0	3.0		
J-K-L	AMT.							
Jam, *Smucker's*	1 tsp.	18	0	4.0	0	0		
Jelly, *Welch's*	2 tsp.	35	0	9.0	0	0		
Kidney beans	1/2 c.	112	.4	20.1	6.5	7.6		
Kiwi fruit, medium	1	46	.3	11.3	2.6	.8		
Lamb loin, lean	4 oz.	229	11.1	0	0	30.2		
Lentils, dry	1/4 c.	70	0	19.0	9.0	8.0		
Lettuce, shredded	1/2 c.	5	.1	1.0	.5	.4		

H
I
J
K
L

Favorite Foods Facts
continued

~FOOD OR BEVERAGE~	AMT.	Calories	Fat grams	Carbs/gms	Fiber/gms	Protein/gms		
M								
Mac.& Cheese, *Kraft*	1 c.	410	18.5	48.0	1.0	11.0		
Maple syrup	1 Tb.	50	0	13.0	0	0		
Margarine	1 Tb.	100	11.0	0	0	0		
Mayonnaise, *Best Fds*	1 Tb.	100	11.0	0	0	0		
Milk, whole	1 c.	150	8.2	11.4	0	8.0		
Milk, non-fat	1 c.	90	0	13.0	0	9.0		
Muffin, English	1	132	1.0	28.7	2.6	4.6		
Mushroom, raw	1/2 c.	9	.2	1.6	.4	.7		
Mustard	1 Tb.	11	1.0	1.0	0	1.0		
N-O	AMT.							
Nectarine, medium	1	67	.6	16.0	2.2	1.3		
Noodles, egg, cooked	1 c.	212	2.4	39.7	1.8	7.6		
Oatmeal, dry	1/2 c.	150	3.0	27.0	4.0	5.0		
Olive oil	1 Tb.	120	14.0	0	0	0		
Onion, raw, chopped	1/2 c.	30	.1	6.9	1.4	.9		
Orange, navel	1	65	.1	16.3	3.4	1.4		
Orange juice	6 oz.	80	0	20.0	.1	0		

Favorite Foods Facts
continued

~FOOD OR BEVERAGE~	AMT.	Calories	Fat grams	Carbs/gms	Fiber/gms	Protein/gms		
P-Q								
Pasta, cooked	1 c.	197	.9	39.7	2.4	6.7		
Peach, fresh	1	37	.1	9.7	1.7	.6		
Peanuts, oil roast	1 oz.	163	13.8	5.3	2.6	7.4		
Peanut butter	2 Tb.	188	16.0	6.6	1.9	7.9		
Pear, fresh	1	98	.7	25.1	4.0	.7		
Peas, fresh, raw	1/2 c.	30	.1	5.4	1.9	2.0		
Pepper, bell, med.	1	20	.1	4.8	1.3	.7		
Pizza, pepperoni	1 slice	253	9.7	27.7	2.2	19.8		
Popcorn,unpopped	1/4c.	110	1.0	26.0	5.0	4.0		
Potato, baked	1	220	.2	51.0	4.8	4.7		
R	AMT.							
Raisins, seedless	1/2 c.	250	0	66.0	4.0	3.0		
Raspberry, red	1/2 c.	31	.3	7.1	4.2	.6		
Refried beans	1/2 c.	134	1.4	23.3	6.7	7.9		
Rice, white, cooked	1 c.	160	.5	38.0	0	3.0		
Rice, brown, cooked	1 c.	166	2.0	37.0	3.0	3.0		

P Q R

Favorite Foods Facts
continued

~FOOD OR BEVERAGE~	AMT.	Calories	Fat grams	Carbs/gms	Fiber/gms	Protein/gms		
S								
Salmon, baked	4 oz.	234	14.0	0	0	25.0		
Salsa, red	2 Tb.	10	0	2.0	0	0		
Sardines in oil, med.	2	50	2.8	0	0	5.9		
Sherbet	1/2 c.	130	1.0	28.0	0	1.0		
Shrimp, large, raw	4	30	.5	.3	0	5.7		
Softdrink, colas, reg.	12 oz.	144	0	38.0	0	0		
Sour cream	1 Tb.	26	2.5	.5	0	.4		
Soy milk	1 c.	79	4.6	4.3	3.9	6.6		
Strawberry, fresh	1/2 c.	23	.3	5.2	1.7	.5		
Sugar, granulated	1 tsp.	15	0	4.0	0	0		
T	AMT.							
Tofu, raw, firm	1/2 c.	183	11.0	5.4	2.9	19.9		
Tomato	1	26	.4	5.7	1.4	1.0		
Tomato juice	6 oz.	32	.1	7.7	.7	1.4		
Tortilla, corn, small	1	40	.5	8.0	1.0	1.0		
Tuna, canned/water	2 oz.	60	.5	0	0	12.0		
Turkey, light meat	4 oz.	178	3.7	0	0	33.9		

Favorite Foods Facts
continued

~FOOD OR BEVERAGE~	AMT.	Calories	Fat grams	Carbs/gms	Fiber/gms	Protein/gms		
U-V-W								
V-8 vegetable juice	6 oz.	35	0	8.0	1.0	1.0		
Vienna sausage	1 oz.	69	7.0	2.0	0	3.0		
Waffle, *Eggo*	1	120	5.0	16.0	0	3.0		
Walnut halves	1 c.	642	61.9	18.3	4.8	14.3		
Watermelon, diced	1/2 c.	25	.3	5.7	.4	.5		
Wheat germ	1 oz.	103	3.4	12.3	3.3	9.3		
Wine, dry, table	1 oz.	25	0	1.2	0	0		
X-Y-Z	AMT.							
Yam, baked/boiled	1/2 c.	79	.1	18.8	2.7	1.0		
Yams, canned	1/2 c.	90	0	20.0	2.0	2.0		
Yogurt, plain, lowfat	1 c.	150	4.0	17.0	0	12.0		
Yogurt, frozen, van.	1/2 c.	110	3.0	19.0	0	3.0		
Zucchini, raw-sliced	1/2 c.	9	.1	1.9	.8	.8		

U
V
W
X
Y
Z

~Graph Records~

A visual way to chart your progress

Range														
Day # or Date →														

This chart :

Range														
Day # or Date →														

This chart :

A visual way to chart your progress

Range									
Day # or Date ↑									

This chart :

Range									
Day # or Date ↑									

This chart :

~*Weekly Progress*~

DATES:					
Weight					
Cholesterol Level					
Blood Pressure					
MEASUREMENTS:					
Chest					
Waist					
Hips					
Neck					
Upper Arms					
Thighs					
Calves					

DATES:					
Weight					
Cholesterol Level					
Blood Pressure					
MEASUREMENTS:					
Chest					
Waist					
Hips					
Neck					
Upper Arms					
Thighs					
Calves					

DATES:					
Weight					
Cholesterol Level					
Blood Pressure					
MEASUREMENTS:					
Chest					
Waist					
Hips					
Neck					
Upper Arms					
Thighs					
Calves					

2012

January						
S	M	T	W	T	F	S
1	2	3	4	5	6	7
8	9	10	11	12	13	14
15	16	17	18	19	20	21
22	23	24	25	26	27	28
29	30	31				

February						
S	M	T	W	T	F	S
			1	2	3	4
5	6	7	8	9	10	11
12	13	14	15	16	17	18
19	20	21	22	23	24	25
26	27	28	29			

March						
S	M	T	W	T	F	S
				1	2	3
4	5	6	7	8	9	10
11	12	13	14	15	16	17
18	19	20	21	22	23	24
25	26	27	28	29	30	31

April						
S	M	T	W	T	F	S
1	2	3	4	5	6	7
8	9	10	11	12	13	14
15	16	17	18	19	20	21
22	23	24	25	26	27	28
29	30					

May						
S	M	T	W	T	F	S
		1	2	3	4	5
6	7	8	9	10	11	12
13	14	15	16	17	18	19
20	21	22	23	24	25	26
27	28	29	30	31		

June						
S	M	T	W	T	F	S
					1	2
3	4	5	6	7	8	9
10	11	12	13	14	15	16
17	18	19	20	21	22	23
24	25	26	27	28	29	30

July						
S	M	T	W	T	F	S
1	2	3	4	5	6	7
8	9	10	11	12	13	14
15	16	17	18	19	20	21
22	23	24	25	26	27	28
29	30	31				

August						
S	M	T	W	T	F	S
			1	2	3	4
5	6	7	8	9	10	11
12	13	14	15	16	17	18
19	20	21	22	23	24	25
26	27	28	29	30	31	

September						
S	M	T	W	T	F	S
						1
2	3	4	5	6	7	8
9	10	11	12	13	14	15
16	17	18	19	20	21	22
23	24	25	26	27	28	29
30						

October						
S	M	T	W	T	F	S
	1	2	3	4	5	6
7	8	9	10	11	12	13
14	15	16	17	18	19	20
21	22	23	24	25	26	27
28	29	30	31			

November						
S	M	T	W	T	F	S
				1	2	3
4	5	6	7	8	9	10
11	12	13	14	15	16	17
18	19	20	21	22	23	24
25	26	27	28	29	30	

December						
S	M	T	W	T	F	S
						1
2	3	4	5	6	7	8
9	10	11	12	13	14	15
16	17	18	19	20	21	22
23	24	25	26	27	28	29
30	31					

2013

January						
S	M	T	W	T	F	S
		1	2	3	4	5
6	7	8	9	10	11	12
13	14	15	16	17	18	19
20	21	22	23	24	25	26
27	28	29	30	31		

February						
S	M	T	W	T	F	S
					1	2
3	4	5	6	7	8	9
10	11	12	13	14	15	16
17	18	19	20	21	22	23
24	25	26	27	28		

March						
S	M	T	W	T	F	S
					1	2
3	4	5	6	7	8	9
10	11	12	13	14	15	16
17	18	19	20	21	22	23
24	25	26	27	28	29	30
31						

April						
S	M	T	W	T	F	S
	1	2	3	4	5	6
7	8	9	10	11	12	13
14	15	16	17	18	19	20
21	22	23	24	25	26	27
28	29	30				

May						
S	M	T	W	T	F	S
			1	2	3	4
5	6	7	8	9	10	11
12	13	14	15	16	17	18
19	20	21	22	23	24	25
26	27	28	29	30	31	

June						
S	M	T	W	T	F	S
						1
2	3	4	5	6	7	8
9	10	11	12	13	14	15
16	17	18	19	20	21	22
23	24	25	26	27	28	29
30						

July						
S	M	T	W	T	F	S
	1	2	3	4	5	6
7	8	9	10	11	12	13
14	15	16	17	18	19	20
21	22	23	24	25	26	27
28	29	30	31			

August						
S	M	T	W	T	F	S
				1	2	3
4	5	6	7	8	9	10
11	12	13	14	15	16	17
18	19	20	21	22	23	24
25	26	27	28	29	30	31

September						
S	M	T	W	T	F	S
1	2	3	4	5	6	7
8	9	10	11	12	13	14
15	16	17	18	19	20	21
22	23	24	25	26	27	28
29	30					

October						
S	M	T	W	T	F	S
		1	2	3	4	5
6	7	8	9	10	11	12
13	14	15	16	17	18	19
20	21	22	23	24	25	26
27	28	29	30	31		

November						
S	M	T	W	T	F	S
					1	2
3	4	5	6	7	8	9
10	11	12	13	14	15	16
17	18	19	20	21	22	23
24	25	26	27	28	29	30

December						
S	M	T	W	T	F	S
1	2	3	4	5	6	7
8	9	10	11	12	13	14
15	16	17	18	19	20	21
22	23	24	25	26	27	28
29	30	31				

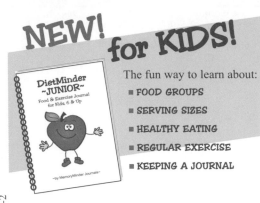
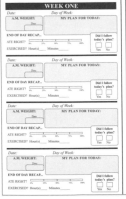

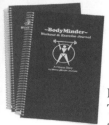

~BodyMinder~
Workout & Exercise Journal
A Fitness Diary

Whether you workout regularly or are just beginning, the BodyMinder can help you stay on track and motivated. This handy journal has become a favorite with fitness buffs at the gym, at home, or anywhere their activities take them. Good for *all* types of exercise, from weight training to aerobics to sporting activities. There's a section for meals, too.

BodyMinder Daily Pages

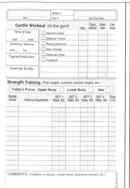

ISBN# 978-0-9637968-4-4

Record:

- Starting statistics
- Weekly plans
- Games
- Daily workout details such as reps, sets, times, equipment, settings
- More details including other exercise, meals, food counts, vitamins, etc.

- Goals
- Progress
- Expenses

"See your goals become reality!"

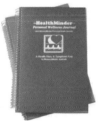

A.K.A.
MemoryMinder
Personal Health Journal

~HealthMinder~
Personal Wellness Journal
Health Diary & Symptoms Log

The HealthMinder makes it easy to record all the details of day-to-day health. It takes just moments to record conditions including pain or other symptoms from head-to-toe. Also track vitamins/medications, diet/exercise, even the weather. Can be used every day or simply whenever changes occur. Discover patterns, track progress, take control of your health!

HealthMinder Daily Pages

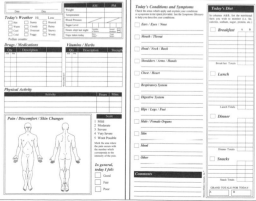

ISBN# 978-0-9637968-7-5

Record:

- Vitamins/herbs
- Medications
- Physical activity
- Allergies
- Blood pressure
- Skin changes
- Symptoms
- Flare-ups
- Sleep habits

- Meals
- Mood
- Pain
- Tests
- Notes
- And more!

"Take an active role in your healthcare!"

To order additional journals...

Mail this order form with your check or money order to:

MemoryMinder Journals

PO Box 23108 • Eugene, OR 97402-0425

(Please allow 1-2 weeks for delivery)

For Visa/Mastercard orders call 1(800) 888-3392 or (541)342-2300

For more information or quotes on large quantities,

call or visit our website,

www.memoryminder.com

SAVE!
When you order
more than one,
deduct $2 per
journal!

- ✂ - - -

DietMinder *Personal Food & Fitness Journal*

Color and Quantity: *Record your meals and more!*

Forest Green_____ Dark Purple_____ @ **$14.95** each = $_____

BodyMinder *Workout & Exercise Journal*

Color and Quantity: *Log your workouts and diet, too!*

Black_____ Burgundy_____ @ **$14.95** each = $_____

HealthMinder *Personal Wellness Journal*

Color and Quantity: *Track your health the easy way!*

Navy_____ Red_____ @ **$14.95** each = $_____

MaintenanceMinder *Daily Weigh-In Journal*

Color and Quantity: *You took it off, now keep it off!*

Deep Brown_____ Ivory_____ @ **$16.95** each = $_____

DietMinder JUNIOR *Journal for Kids 6 & Up*

Quantity_____ *Start Early-Stay Healthy!* @ **$10.95** each = $_____

*Discount...$2 off each book when ordering 2 or more: (minus) ($_____)

Subtotal $_____

Shipping/Handling: add $4.95 for the first book = $____4.95____

...plus $1.00 for each additional book = $_____

Total (Payment enclosed) = $

Please circle where you learned about **MemoryMinder** *Journals:*

*Magazine   Store   Friend   Internet   Other*_____

Name_____Phone (_____)_____

Required on all mail orders.

Company/organization_____

Mailing Address_____

City_____St_____Zip_____

ISBN# 978-0-9637968-3-7